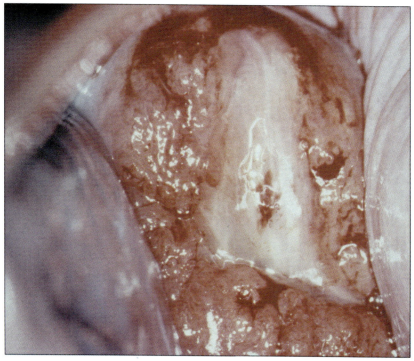

Colposcopic photograph of cervix cleaned with cotton wool demonstrating acute haemorrhagic chlamydial cervicitis. Presenting symptoms:- post coital/intermenstrual bleeding.

International Handbook of Chlamydia

This book is due for return on or before the last date shown below.

30. MAR 2011		

International Handbook of Chlamydia

Edited by

Dr TR Moss
*Doncaster Royal Infirmary,
Doncaster, England*

Acknowledgement
The editor would like to thank Mrs Joan Pleasance
for her patience and professionalism.

ISBN 1 899015 43 4

Printed in the United Kingdom by Polestar Wheatons Ltd, Exeter, UK

Contents

Foreword

In recent years bacterial sexually transmitted diseases (STD) have been overshadowed by the growing epidemic of viral STDs, in particular HIV. In addition, the declining prevalence of some bacterial infections in the last 20 years may have suggested that these agents were diseases of the past, of diminishing importance and of limited interest outside specialist care. This has never been the case with chlamydial genital infections and it is timely that we should review their importance, particularly in the light of recent developments.

Following the isolation of *Chlamydia trachomatis* from genital secretions in the late 1950s the importance of particular serovars has been increasingly recognised. Early work identified *C. trachomatis* as the cause of much symptomatic genital disease and as the putative cause of fallopian tube disease through both direct and indirect mechanisms. Key work in the seventies identified genital *C. trachomatis* as the likely cause of most secondary infertility in the developed world – emphasising the importance of establishing its control as a public health goal. Making the arguments for this and demonstrating the benefits of a major screening and treatment programme for this agent has not been easy.

Epidemiological work, initially within STD treatment clinics, has shown that most *C. trachomatis* infection is silent in both females and males. Work outside these settings in the community has confirmed this finding showing high levels of prevalence of silent infection in women, particularly in higher risk groups. Interventions targeted at identifying and treating infection in some of these groups alone has led to a limited level of success in the prevention of early complications of missed infection. However, the prevalence of Chlamydia within the community has shown no decline. It would therefore appear that genital *C. trachomatis* infection is hyperendic in the developed world, and that limited interventions within high-risk groups will not lead to its control. The challenge in recent years has been to show that a comprehensive screening programme is practical, acceptable to patients and cost-effective.

A number of health providers had already acted before such data were available and their experience has helped inform us of decisions we may now be faced with. Mass screening and treatment programmes in Northern Europe have demonstrated that regular investigation of sexually active women was indeed followed by a reduction in chlamydial prevalence. Such early programmes utilised sample collection and processing methodologies that were far from perfect but despite these weaknesses considerable progress has been made in controlling chlamydial disease. This reduction has been accompanied by a much larger decline in tubal disease within these countries. Such indirect evidence offered support to the concept that intervention programmes are cost effective.

Recently, healthcare providers in North America have instigated controlled intervention studies of screening and treatment for chlamydial infections. These projects have looked in detail at the differing expenses of managing chlamydial disease. The majority of the expenses within screening programmes are the costs in clinical time in gathering specimens and initiating contact tracing. Even so, cost benefit-analyses have clearly shown that screening and effective treatment are highly cost effective within managed healthcare systems.

Modelling of different screening strategies demonstrates that the final set point for chlamydial prevalence after a number of years of implementation is a function of the sensitivity of a screening test and its take up. The recent development of new, non-invasive, highly sensitive, molecular technology-based methods for chlamydial identification have been piloted. These tests can use patient gathered samples such as urine. The exact place of these tests and the feasibility of their usage is yet to be clearly established. However, preliminary results from pilot community-based screening projects are highly encouraging showing that these methods are practical, acceptable to patients and yield levels of chlamydial infection similar to those in STD clinic attendees.

Contact tracing of partners has always been a central pillar of STD management and control. A debate is currently taking place as to whether a traditional approach to contact tracing is possible if extensive screening programmes are initiated. The international experience suggests that in some settings some of the responsibility may be passed to primary care – however this may not be appropriate in all settings and the results of different strategies of contact tracing, being trialed within pilot programmes, are eagerly awaited.

A number of infectious agents have recently been identified as key to the development and maintenance of chronic medical conditions. There has been considerable interest in the role of both *Chlamydia pneumoniae* and CMV in the development of atherosclerosis. Although early antibiotic intervention studies have been disappointing, interest in *C. pneumoniae* as a cofactor for cardiovascular disease is still being actively researched and debated.

Great progress has been made during the late 20th century in decreasing the tragedy of avoidable blindness following trachoma. Whilst the International Handbook has concentrated on human genital infection with *C. trachomatis* the exciting developments in morbidity due to, or possibly resulting from other chlamydial agents has clearly justified specific chapters relating to non-genital chlamydial disease.

The objective of this text has been to increase knowledge, awareness and understanding of disease due to chlamydial pathogens. It has also been intended to promote a wider debate and to provoke argument when incomplete understanding clearly exists. Hypothesis, future speculation and controversy have been encouraged rather than avoided. We have much to learn.

Dr Raj Patel
Department of Genito Urinary Medicine,
Royal South Hants Hospital, Southampton, UK

Preface

During November 1999 the Department of Microbiology at this hospital met to discuss the application of new diagnostic techniques in the identification and management of human genital chlamydial infections.

At very short notice I was asked to Chair the meeting based on the purpose of my original appointment at this hospital (1980), which was to develop (in collaboration with Microbiology) a clinical diagnostic service for genital chlamydial infections.

The success of that endeavour was largely due to one of our Laboratory Scientists, the late Stephen Riddington, whose contribution merits specific recognition.

Following this meeting I was approached by Dr Jane Sefton of Roche Diagnostics, and asked – (having regard for the recently published UK National Guidelines on managing genital chlamydial infection together with the proposed pilot population screening projects) – was there a place for a monograph covering clinical and diagnostic aspects of chlamydial infection?

The existence of this book clearly identifies my response to her concept.

Our aim has been to identify areas of debate and controversy as well as to acknowledge the limitations in our current knowledge and understanding of these diseases.

The opportunity has been given for authors to identify hopes and aspirations for the future. It was considered important that genital chlamydial infections are seen not only in terms of acute sexually transmitted disease, but also the complexity of disease spectrum should be discussed. Contributors were asked to address those problems which are particularly related to subacute and chronic disease; and to consider the concept of latency. A further concern was to review aspects of non-genital human chlamydial infection.

In recent broadcasts such phrases as "we can screen for cancer of the cervix and breast; we could screen for prostate cancer and *even Chlamydia*" identify that both in professional and in public perception chlamydial diseases may be trivialised.

This spectrum of diseases challenges such trivialisation. Future generations of clinicians and scientists have the opportunity to contribute to the identification, care, control and prevention of one of the world's most prevalent and important group of infectious diseases.

Both public and professionals may need reminding that women still die from the complications of genital chlamydial disease via ruptured ectopic pregnancy, and such deaths occur in all developed healthcare systems.

The cost (in terms of individual suffering to women) of a lifetime of pelvic pain, infertility and sexual disability is profound.

The enormous avoidable financial costs to health service provision are, understandably driving forward improvements in clinical services.

This book identifies that much has been achieved during the last half of the twentieth century. Clearly, we can and must do better in the twenty-first century. Success is anticipated.

Dr TR Moss
Consultant Physician/Clinical Director,
Genito-Urinary Medicine, Doncaster Royal Infirmary, Doncaster, UK

CHAPTER 1

Epidemiology

Ian Simms
PHLS Communicable Disease Surveillance Centre, London, UK

INTRODUCTION

Chlamydia trachomatis is a bacterial infection of global public health significance. It is associated with trachoma (serovars A, B, B_1 and C), lymphogranuloma venereum (serovars L_1, L_2 and L_3) and genital infection (serovars D to K). Genital *C. trachomatis* infection can cause pelvic inflammatory disease (PID) and represents a major public health problem to the reproductive health of women in developed and developing countries. The World Health Organization estimates that 89 million new cases of genital *C. trachomatis* infection occur each year (**Table 1**)[1]. Cataract, glaucoma and trachoma are the three commonest causes of blindness worldwide. Trachoma affects 150 million people, of whom 6 million are blind. Lymphogranuloma venereum (LGV) also has a global distribution, but is uncommon in industrialised countries and its prevalence is unknown.

Trachoma, LGV and genital *C. trachomatis* infection pose contrasting public health challenges. Trachoma, a fomite, was a leading cause of blindness in Europe but disappeared during the early twentieth century, eliminated as much by improved personal hygiene, sanitation and reduced housing occupancy as improved intervention. Chlamydial ophthalmia neonatorum and adult chlamydial eye infections, resulting from autoinoculation with genital secretions, still occur in Europe but are self-limiting and never progress to trachoma. *C. trachomatis* is easily treated and the WHO aims to eliminate trachoma blindness by 2020 although, since it is a disease of poverty, this is dependent on economic growth as well as improved healthcare. In contrast,

Table 1. Estimated number of new cases, prevalence and incidence of genital *C. trachomatis* infection between ages 15 and 49, by sex and United Nation global region: 1995[1]

Region	New cases (million)		Prevalence (%)		Incidence (per 1000)	
	Males	Females	Males	Females	Males	Females
North America	1.64	2.34	0.8	2.7	21.46	30.73
Western Europe	2.30	3.20	0.8	2.7	21.46	30.73
Australasia	0.12	0.17	0.8	2.7	21.46	30.73
Latin America & Caribbean	5.01	5.12	2.5	4.0	40.03	40.77
Sub-Saharan Africa	6.96	8.44	4.8	7.1	55.04	65.95
North Africa & Middle East	1.67	1.28	1.2	1.7	19.93	16.29
Eastern Europe & Central Asia	2.15	2.92	1.7	3.7	27.29	37.09
East Asia & Pacific	2.70	2.63	0.4	0.7	6.53	6.75
South & South East Asia	20.20	20.28	3.7	4.9	41.65	44.32
Overall	42.75	46.38	–	–	–	–

genital *C. trachomatis* infection and LGV will not be eliminated in the foreseeable future as both are sexually transmitted infections (STI) with complex epidemiologies.

Chlamydial research has been guided by developments in diagnostic techniques. Cheap diagnostic tests with good specificity and sensitivity became available in the mid-1980's, and clinical and epidemiological studies quickly established the importance of genital *C. trachomatis* infection and its sequelae. Surveillance information is now available for countries in Europe, North America and the developing world, data that have been used as an evidence base for clinical practice, public health action, and control and intervention strategies. This chapter presents an overview of the epidemiology of genital *C. trachomatis* infection and explores the increasing importance of epidemiological methods and behavioural studies to chlamydial research.

PREVALENCE, INCIDENCE AND DISEASE BURDEN

Geographically, the majority of genital *C. trachomatis* infections are found in the developing world reflecting provision and access to healthcare, health seeking behaviour and the global population distribution (**Table 1**). Highest prevalences are in sub-Saharan Africa, lowest in East Asia and the Pacific.

However, these estimates are biased due to the quality and quantity of the available surveillance data. Many countries do not have national surveillance data and, where prevalence studies have been undertaken, these have generally been derived from high risk groups such as STD clinic attenders. A further source of bias is the high level of asymptomatic infection. Up to 70% of infections in women and 50% of infections in men are asymptomatic and thus do not seek treatment and this pool of asymptomatic infection is unlikely to be represented in surveillance datasets. However, although biased, these estimates illustrate the global importance of genital *C. trachomatis* infection.

Genital *C. trachomatis* infection is of public health importance because it can lead to pelvic inflammatory disease (PID). PID can be caused by genital mycoplasmas, endogenous vaginal flora (anaerobic and aerobic bacteria), aerobic streptococci, *Mycobacterium tuberculosis*, and STIs such as *C. trachomatis* or *Neisseria gonorrhoeae*. However, genital *C. trachomatis* infection is considered the dominant cause of PID in developed countries. Between 10% and 40% of *C. trachomatis* cases develop PID[2]. Sequelae of PID include ectopic pregnancy, tubal factor infertility and chronic pelvic pain, PID has also been associated with increased risk of ovarian cancer[3,4]. The risk of developing sequelae is dependent on the number of PID episodes: the risk of ectopic pregnancy and infertility increases after one PID episode (odds ratio=6) and again after two episodes (OR=17)[5].

Infertility related to genital *C. trachomatis* infection is of public health importance in sub-Saharan Africa and the treatment of infection and associated sequelae absorb a sizeable part of healthcare resources in developing countries. In developed countries costs have increased substantially since the development of assisted reproduction techniques, such as *in vitro* fertilisation. In 1992, the cost of a subfertility service in one health district in England and Wales with a population of 46 000 women aged 20 to 44 years was estimated to be £0.88 million, a national total of £75 million[6]. Of this cost, 20% (£14 million) was likely to be associated with genital *C. trachomatis* infection and could have been prevented. PID accounts for 94% of morbidity in women associated with STIs (including HIV) in established market economies. Indeed, the burden of PID among women, measured in terms of disability adjusted life years, was higher than the burden of disease associated with HIV among men. In terms of economic cost, both PID and its sequelae are expensive to individuals, healthcare services and economies. In the USA, direct and indirect costs associated with PID and its sequelae have been projected to exceed $10 billion by the year 2000[7]. However, these studies

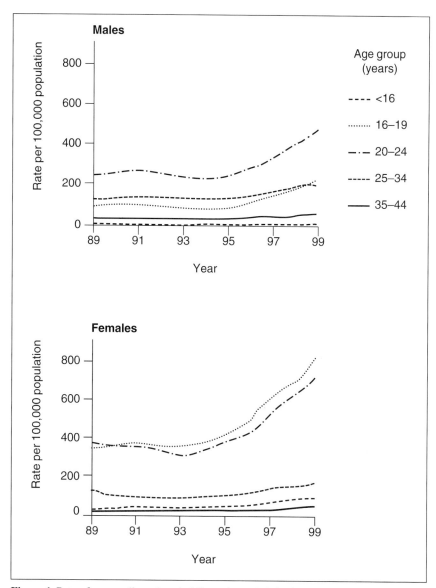

Figure 1. Rate of uncomplicated genital *C. trachomatis* infection by age group, England and Wales: 1989 to 1999

may be inaccurate as the incidence and prevalence of PID are unknown.

Although national surveillance is now undertaken in most countries, few have collected data for more than a decade and, where available, it is usually restricted to laboratory reports or attendences at STD clinics. Trends in surveillance data should be interpreted with caution as they can be influenced by a number of factors such as changes in testing policy, clinical practice, the availability and accuracy of diagnostic tests, access to healthcare and the prevalence of asymptomatic infection. In addition, the limited number of parameters collected restricts interpretation. For example, data for England and Wales have been collected since 1988 but only include information on gender, age group and geographic location and consequently can only show broad trends over time (**Figure 1**). The increases seen in England and Wales during the past decade probably reflect increased public and professional awareness to genital *C. trachomatis* infection and increased testing. As in many other countries, the dataset derived from STD clinics in England and Wales needs to be developed to meet the increased need for detailed, timely surveillance data. STI epidemiology is driven by a complex mixture of behavioural, microbiological and demographic factors and these need to be included in surveillance systems. Surveillance also needs to be multi-faceted and include assessment of sexual ill-health, behaviour and service data as these data play a key role in establishing an evidence base to plan, monitor, audit and evaluate programmes intended to improve sexual health.

In recent years, studies in various clinical settings have been undertaken to investigate the prevalence of infection, evaluate testing methodologies and assess service delivery. In England and Wales, studies carried out in selected population groups indicate prevalences of 2% to 12%: higher prevalences were seen in attenders at STD and termination of pregnancy clinics, lower prevalences in primary care. A large evidence base is now available but the data should be treated with caution. Studies undertaken have generally been based on small numbers, confined to healthcare attender populations and have included a wide range of sampling and testing methodologies. The range of testing methodologies represents a particular problem because the sensitivity and specificity varies between testing strategies and over time. This will have influenced both the number of positive and false positive cases detected. These limitations suggest that detected prevalences are not absolute levels and consequently interpretation is difficult, as are comparisons between studies and extrapolation of findings to the wider population.

WHO IS AT RISK?

Risk factor studies can identify population subgroups at increased risk of genital *C. trachomatis* infection, and be used to initiate timely, effective, intervention and help formulate health education strategies. Incidence is influenced by a complex interaction of demographic and behavioural factors. Aspects of sexual behaviour, such as age at first sexual intercourse, number of lifetime sexual partners, frequency of partner change and unsafe sex, are key determinants of STI transmission. Age at first sexual intercourse and the number of lifetime sexual partners are known to vary with marital status, cohabitation and socio-economic group. Young people are behaviourally vulnerable to STI acquisition as they generally have higher numbers of sexual partners and a higher frequency of partner change than older age groups[8]. In addition, young people may be at particular risk of re-infection as they may not have the skills and confidence to negotiate safer sex. These factors are reflected in the high chlamydial incidence seen in the 16 to 24 year age group, peaking younger in females than males (**Figure 1**). Studies on specific populations have shown that factors such as being unmarried, the use of non-barrier contraceptives (or no contraception), a higher frequency of partner change, having concurrent partners and lower socio-economic status are associated with higher chlamydial incidence.

A large number of risk factor studies have been published from various countries, but invariably these have been undertaken in specific clinical settings and are insufficient to allow detailed analyses. The relationship between sexual behaviour and STI prevalence has been little studied in general population samples. Sexual behaviour varies between societies, individuals and during an individual's lifetime. The interaction between the core group (people who have large numbers of sexual partners, concurrent partners and frequent partner change) and the rest of the population, is important to STI transmission. The investigation of sexual networks, the basis of interactions between the core and the rest of the population, is a key area of research. Behavioural, demographic and morbidity surveillance at the individual level provides more precise estimates of risk factors associated with genital *C. trachomatis* infection. The National Survey of Sexual Attitudes and Lifestyles (NATSSAL) 1990/91, was the first UK survey of sexual behaviour and included an extensive range of data on partnerships, sexual practice, condom use, sexuality and risk reduction practices[8]. Similar studies have been undertaken in other countries. The 2000/1 survey includes an assessment of the prevalence of genital *C. trachomatis* infection and associated demographic and behavioural risk factors.

EPIDEMIOLOGY OF PELVIC INFLAMMATORY DISEASE (PID)

Little is known of PID epidemiology: the burden of disease and associated risk factors are poorly understood but need to be investigated to inform public health action and clinical practice. Although a substantial burden of PID is thought to exist in many countries, surveillance data are only available for a few European countries, mostly in Scandinavia. Epidemics of *C. trachomatis* and *N. gonorrhoeae* are followed by a secondary PID epidemic and tertiary epidemics of ectopic pregnancy and tubal factor infertility. In England and Wales, variations in gonorrhoea cases seen in STD clinics and hospital inpatient attendances for PID and ectopic pregnancy have followed this pattern (**Figure 2**). Interpretation is, however, difficult as there are a number of gaps in reporting. The lack of surveillance data also makes it difficult to assess the contribution of genital *C. trachomatis* infection to the PID and ectopic pregnancy epidemics. Hospital

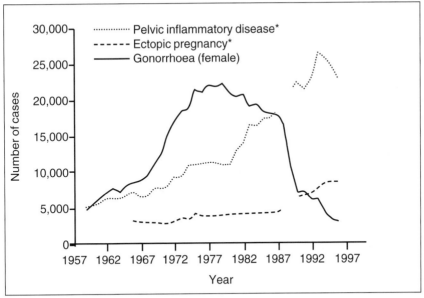

Figure 2. Gonorrhoea, pelvic inflammatory disease and ectopic pregnancy, England and Wales: 1957 to 1997

* Hospital inpatient collection method changed after 1985: no data available for 1986 and 1987. Ectopic pregnancy data were not available before 1964.

in-patient data consist of acute cases, women experiencing recurrent chronic pain and long-term reproductive health problems associated with PID. Consequently these data underestimate the true reservoir of PID in the general population. In fact data from primary care suggest that 165,000 cases occur every year in reproductive age women, a prevalence of 1.7% in England and Wales.

Risk factors for PID development are closely associated with those of STI acquisition. High PID rates in women aged 16 to 24 years may reflect longer duration of chlamydial infection or reduced clearance of chlamydial infection in younger women. This could be due to increased host susceptibility, such as a lower concentration of protective chlamydial antibodies, larger cervical ectopy, and greater permeability of cervical mucus than in older age groups. A number of factors have been associated with PID. IUD insertion and termination of pregnancy have been associated with iatrogenic PID, which occurs when instrumentation facilitates the introduction of micro-organisms into the endometrial cavity. Cigarette smoking has been associated with increased risk of PID. Smoking is thought to either compromise the immune response to infection or the activity of oestrogen. It is also likely that smoking reflects poor health seeking behaviour in lower socio-economic groups. The association between PID and oral contraceptive (OC) use is also complex and incompletely understood. Although OC use has been associated with a 50% decrease in PID in reported studies, it is unclear whether OC use prevents ascending infection or protects against symptomatic infection. Alternatively both cigarette smoking and OC use may simply be confounding factors that reflect higher sexual risk. Douching has been associated with PID as it is thought to alter the microbiological environment of the vagina and flush bacteria into the uterus. However, although douching is common amongst women in the USA, less than 0.25% of UK women report this behaviour. This shows that it is unlikely that douching is an important factor associated with PID in the UK and that it is unwise to extrapolate the findings of risk factor studies between countries as sexual health behaviour and contraceptive practice vary substantially.

CONTROL AND INTERVENTION

Primary prevention, based on education and behavioural change, is fundamental to disease control. Behavioural change, such as the increased use of barrier contraception and delayed sexual debut, in response to HIV and STI health campaigns has been documented in European countries and some have been associated with reduced incidence of symptomatic PID[9-12]. However, in the UK and many other countries, the major obstacle to primary prevention is a low awareness of PID amongst healthcare professionals and the public. Secondary prevention, or the diagnosis and treatment of asymptomatic infection, has been successful in reducing both the prevalence of genital *C. trachomatis* infection and PID. The only randomised controlled trial to look at the effectiveness of genital chlamydial screening indicated that decreases in the prevalence of genital *C. trachomatis* infection brought about reductions in PID prevalence[13]. In the USA, intervention based on screening for genital *C. trachomatis* infection has also reduced the incidence of PID and ectopic pregnancy by more than 50% and 20% respectively[14]. Swedish data also indicate that screening for genital *C. trachomatis* infection rapidly reduces the incidence of ectopic pregnancy amongst 20 to 24 year olds[15]. No study has demonstrated that genital *C. trachomatis* screening can reduce the prevalence of tubal factor infertility.

Surveillance is central to effective, efficient and sustainable intervention. Timely estimates of the prevalence and incidence of infection and sequelae, together with associated risk factors are needed to assess the impact of intervention. If screening is used, estimates of transmission dynamics and the duration of infectiousness will also be required to evaluate the screening interval.

DEVELOPMENTS IN EPIDEMIOLOGICAL RESEARCH

Chlamydial research continues to be guided by developments in diagnostic methods. Over the past decade molecular techniques have been applied to chlamydial diagnostic tests, this has led to the development of tests which combine ease of collection and transport, with high sensitivity and specificity. Molecular techniques have also allowed greater flexibility in study design. Self obtained vaginal and vulval swabs or non-invasive specimens such as urine can be collected in non-clinical settings and mailed for testing. These developments have increased the acceptability of testing to patients and allowed the integration of microbiological and behavioural research methods within large population-based epidemiological studies. Multiplex testing, the simultaneous amplification of several pathogens, such as *C. trachomatis*, *N. gonorrhoeae*, and *Mycoplasma genitalium*, offers low cost testing, and the ability to investigate concurrent infections within population subgroups.

Behavioural research has also evolved and now includes computer-assisted data capture methods such as computer-assisted personal interview and computer-assisted self-interview methods which offer increased response rates and improved disclosure of sensitive sexual behaviours.

CONCLUSIONS

Genital *C. trachomatis* infection is a key global issue facing women's reproductive health. This is a rapidly expanding area of research but for many countries the available data do not provide an accurate view of the epidemiology of either genital *C. trachomatis* infection or the associated burden of disease. This prevents a true realisation of the burden of reproductive morbidity and represents a fundamental gap in our knowledge of STI epidemiology. Epidemiological research is a continuous process that requires the routine collection of behavioural, demographic and laboratory data tailored to the public health needs and priorities of individual countries. However, despite substantial research over the past two decades, we are only just beginning to comprehend the public health impact of this important infection.

REFERENCES

1. Gerbase A, Rowley J, Heymann D, Berkley S, Piot P. (1998). Global prevalence and incidence estimates of selected curable STDs. *Sex Transm Inf* **74:** S12–4.
2. Stamm W, Guinan M, Johnson C, Starcher T, Holmes K, McCormack W. (1984). Effect of treatment regimens for *Neisseria gonorrhoeae* on simultaneous infection with *Chlamydia trachomatis*. *N Engl J Med* **310:** 545–9.
3. Buchan H, Vessey M, Goldacre M, Fairweather J. (1993). Morbidity following pelvic inflammatory disease. *Br J Obstet Gynaecol* **100:** 558–62.
4. Risch H, Howe G. (1995). Pelvic inflammatory disease and the risk of epithelial ovarian cancer. *Cancer Epidemiol Biomarkers Prev* **4:** 447–51.
5. Weström L. (1994). Sexually Transmitted Diseases and Infertility. *Sex Trans Dis* **21:** S32–7.
6. School of Public Health UoL. Effective Health Care: The Management of Subfertility. Leeds *University of Leeds* 1992.
7. Washington A, Katz P. (1991). Cost of and payment source for pelvic inflammatory disease. *JAMA* **226:** 2565–9.
8. Johnson A, Wadsworth J, Wellings K, Field J, Bradshaw S. (1994). Sexual Attitudes and Lifestyles. Oxford. Blackwell Scientific Publications.
9. Wølner-Hanssen P, Eschenbach D, Paavonen J. (1990). Decreased risk of symptomatic chlamydial pelvic inflammatory disease associated with oral contraception use. *JAMA* **263:** 54–9.
10. Evans B, Catchpole M, Heptonstall M, *et al.* (1993). Sexually transmitted diseases and HIV-1 infection among homosexual men in England and Wales. *Br Med J* **306:** 426–8.
11. Weström L. (1988). Decrease in incidence of women treated in hospital for acute salpingitis in Sweden. *Genitourin Med* **64:** 59–63.

12. Coutinho R, Rijsdijk A, van den Hoek J, Leentvaar-Kuijpers A. (1992). Decreasing incidence of PID in Amsterdam. *Genitourin Med* **68:** 353–5.
13. Scholes D, Stergachis A, Heidrich F, Andrilla H, Holmes KK, Stamm W. (1996). Prevention of pelvic inflammatory disease by screening for cervical chlamydial infection. *N Engl J Med* **334:** 1362–6.
14. Hillis S, Nakashima A, Amsterdam L, *et al.* (1995). The impact of a comprehensive chlamydia prevention program in Wisconsin. *Fam Plan Perspect* **27:** 108–111.
15. Egger M, Low N, Smith G, Lindblom B, Herrmann B. (1998). Screening for chlamydia infections and the risk of ectopic pregnancy in a county in Sweden:ecological analysis. *Br Med J* **316:** 1776–80.

CHAPTER 2

Chlamydia trachomatis
– the case for screening

Angela Robinson
Mortimer Market Centre, London, UK

Chlamydia trachomatis is the commonest bacterial sexually transmitted infection in the UK today. The majority of infections are asymptomatic but sequelae are common. These include pelvic inflammatory disease which may result in ectopic pregnancy and infertility, neonatal infections, epididymitis and joint inflammation in men. The direct healthcare costs of management of the complications are high and the human costs, although difficult to quantify, are considerable.

Before embarking on an intervention such as screening, evidence for the effectiveness of this proposed intervention and delivery of health gain is needed. The randomised controlled trial published by Scholes[1] was the first "proof" that selective screening for *C. trachomatis* reduced complications. The incidence of pelvic infection was reduced by more than half in the screened population. Other evidence has been obtained from case studies. In Uppsala, Sweden the number of positive specimens fell annually to reach 40% of 1985 level by 1991 after widespread screening became available in healthcare settings which attracted young people[2]. Pelvic infection rates and number of ectopic pregnancies have subsequently fallen in Sweden which suggests that widespread screening for *C. trachomatis* does reduce these expensive complications. In Wisconsin, a programme of selective screening in family planning clinics was set up in 1985. Selective screening was undertaken on the basis of risk factor analysis. The prevalence fell overall by 53%[3].

SCREENING FOR *CHLAMYDIA TRACHOMATIS* AND THE WILSON JUNGER CRITERIA

Wilson and Junger described eight guidelines to consider when deciding whether screening was an appropriate strategy for disease prevention. The evidence to support the case of screening for *C. trachomatis* is discussed below for each of these guidelines.

The condition should be an important problem

There is no doubt that genital chlamydial infection is very common. The disease affects approximately 10% of women under 25 years. Prevalence data have been reported from various healthcare settings. The most recent data are available from two pilot studies, one in the Wirral and one in Portsmouth, of screening for *C. trachomatis* undertaken in community settings and show higher than expected prevalence rates according to previous reports from various healthcare settings in the United Kingdom[4]. The highest rates are in 16-20 year olds and range from 9-14%. Data collected through genitourinary medicine clinics indicate a rise in prevalence over the past few years. In teenage men cases of chlamydial infection have increased by 23% and amongst women by 20%[5].

Pelvic inflammatory disease (PID) is an important sequela. The most recent UK study suggested that chlamydial infection is implicated in approximately 50% of cases[6]. Although the data on incidence of PID are difficult to collect, acute PID seems to be rising in teenagers. There has been a slight decrease in the late 1980s and early 1990s in other age groups but nothing to compare with Scandinavian countries.

Pelvic infection may lead to more severe morbidity. Compared to controls with no evidence of pelvic infection, women with a previous history of pelvic infection have ten times the risk of non-specific abdominal pain, four times the risk of "gynaecological" pain, ten times the risk of having an ectopic pregnancy and an eight fold risk of having a subsequent hysterectomy[7].

Women with PID also have a substantially increased incidence of infertility. Asymptomatic pelvic infection may also lead to subsequent tubal infertility with no known clinical episode of PID. *C. trachomatis* is the commonest preventable cause of tubal infertility. The proportion of infertility due to tubal damage ranges from 14-20% and chlamydial infection is implicated in 90% of tubal infertility[8,9].

The natural history of the condition should be adequately understood
Some information is known about the natural history of infection. Clearance of the infection without treatment does occur, but the exact proportion is unknown. The assumption used was 20% in the model developed by DoH Expert Advisory Group[10]. The infection is likely to be transmitted to a sexual partner in up to 80% of cases. It is understood less well why some people develop symptoms whilst others do not. Similarly some women develop symptomatic pelvic infection whereas others have 'silent' tubal infection. Some advances have been made in the immunology of genital chlamydial infection. Following infection some immunity is induced. High titres of heat shock protein have been shown to be associated with pelvic inflammatory disease, tubal infertility and a lower take-home baby rate following *in vitro* fertilisation[11].

There must be a recognisable latent or early symptomatic stage
Asymptomatic chlamydial infection is very common and may be more than the quoted data of 50% in men and 70% in women which are derived predominantly from information obtained through genito-urinary medicine clinics. It may be as high as 90% in men[12]. Symptoms may be transient and therefore infected individuals are less likely to come forward for testing in appropriate healthcare settings.

There should be an accepted and effective treatment for people with recognised disease
Treatment of chlamydial infections is safe and effective with appropriate antibiotics. Several regimens exist and research on the acceptability and cost-effectiveness of these different options is required. Compliance may be an important factor in effectiveness of treatment. Choice of therapy may also be influenced by pregnancy and type of contraception used.

Facilities for diagnosis and treatment should be available
Tests for *C. trachomatis* are routinely undertaken on all patients attending genitourinary medicine services. Testing for *C. trachomatis* is recommended before instrumentation of the cervix. Strong evidence exists for testing all attendees at termination of pregnancy clinics[13]; the evidence for screening before procedures requiring other instrumentation are not so strong apart from pre-IUD fitting[14]. Facilities for diagnosis and treatment are readily available in hospitals and primary healthcare settings although not used optimally at present.

With appropriate professional and public education, healthcare settings could be developed to provide access for screening sexually active women and men for genital chlamydial infection. There are networks of Community Family Planning Clinics and general practitioners that see the target groups. Training of clinicians and provision of resources are essential forerunners to expanding screening. Enhancing present diagnostic testing for *C. trachomatis* in other hospital specialities such as Urology, Accident and Emergency, Obstetrics and Gynaecology (including antenatal and colposcopy) Clinics is feasible. The offering of testing as part of the diagnostic process for patients who may have symptoms attributable to *C. trachomatis* should be encouraged irrespective of any additional initiatives to screen asymptomatic patients.

There are obvious logistical difficulties to overcome with regard to offering widespread chlamydial testing in a number of healthcare settings.

Treatment is readily available in most of these settings, Family Planning Clinics being a notable exception. However with appropriate links and collaboration, management of *C. trachomatis* can be undertaken in other settings, if this cannot be provided to the documented standards of care required, where screening is undertaken.

There should be a suitable test or examination available
The Scandinavian experience suggests that even using lower sensitivity tests such as culture and enzyme immuno-assay, together with other measures, screening for chlamydial infection was an effective intervention to decrease prevalence and complications[15]. The development of sensitive DNA amplification tests which can be used on samples obtained non-invasively makes the introduction of screening even more feasible. There are choices of samples that can be collected from women; urine samples, although convenient for the patient, require a "cold-chain" from site of test to laboratory. Handling time by laboratory staff is longer which makes urine specimens more costly to test. In addition there are problems with inhibitors that can reduce sensitivity. A cheaper, alternative specimen for women is a self-taken vaginal swab that has proved to be as sensitive as doctor-taken cervical specimens. This affords better sensitivity than urine specimens[16]. This is more fully discussed in chapter 3. A urine sample for men is easily obtained but there may be other possible specimens, such as meatal swabs, which would avoid the transportation problems of urine samples.

The test or examination should be acceptable to both public and professionals

As *C. trachomatis* is a sexually transmitted infection, management involves at least one other person. To avoid re-infection it is vital that the partner or partners of identified positives are tested and treated as part of the overall strategy.

Within genitourinary medicine clinics, testing, partner notification for testing and treatment of sexually transmitted infections have proved highly acceptable. It is possible that in other healthcare settings where discussion of sexual partnerships may come unexpectedly, issues which need to be raised may be unacceptable to some patients. Appropriate public education to highlight the importance of chlamydial infections may well counterbalance the potential problems of identifying a sexually transmitted infection. However clinicians need to recognise the difficulties which ensue when discussing infections in the context of sexual relationships.

There should be an agreed policy on whom to treat as patients, including management of cases with equivocal results

Genitourinary medicine clinics have an appropriate infrastructure for follow-up of patients, partner notification and management of partners. There are agreed standards to which these aspects of management are practised. This package of care is more difficult to deliver in other healthcare settings. There are several options of care provision; devolving some aspects of management within healthcare settings where screening is undertaken; developing appropriate referral mechanisms through care pathways. Local arrangements, including a policy on management of patients with equivocal results, need to be in place before embarking on any screening programme.

Measuring the success of any screening strategy relies upon appropriate data collection. Genitourinary medicine departments presently play a key role together with public health departments in gathering information about the epidemiology of sexually transmitted infections locally. These departments need to assess the impact of interventions such as screening.

In addition there are two other criteria to consider: screening interval and costs.

SCREENING INTERVAL AND REINFECTION

Firstly screening should be a continuous process. Little is known about re-infection rates in the United Kingdom. However work undertaken in the USA suggests that a significant proportion of patients identified with chlamydial infection become re-infected within 6 months[17]. Also adolescents who at initial screening have a negative result are at high risk of becoming infected. In a recently reported postal follow-up survey undertaken in Denmark, the re-infection rate for genital chlamydial infection was 30%[18]. Efforts must be directed at accessing partners, who have a high prevalence of chlamydial infection and are the most likely source of re-infection.

Risks for being re-infected with *C. trachomatis* depend on sexual behaviour with regard to both number of partners and unprotected sexual intercourse particularly with a partner who did not receive treatment following the initial diagnosis. Further research is needed to establish re-infection rates but the screening interval will have a great impact on the cost of screening as an intervention. With recent data suggesting high re-infection rates in adolescents and high re-acquisition rates in patients known to have had chlamydial infection, people identified with chlamydial infection would appear to be an important target group for re-screening. Awareness of the high re-infection risk is mandatory for any educational initiative.

COSTS OF CHLAMYDIAL INFECTION

In the United States, the estimate of direct and indirect costs of infection with *C. trachomatis*, including complications, was $13,000 per 1000 of the population aged 16-64 years[19,20]. When applied to the UK population the total cost estimated is over £200 million per annum.

Clearly the cost of early diagnosis and treatment should be balanced in economic terms in relation to total expenditure on medical care. Several cost effective analyses have been undertaken. A major drawback in all models is the need to make assumptions (probability estimates) about likelihood of development of complications, re-infection rates, uptake of screening in men and screening intervals. However there is consensus that above prevalence rates of 4-6%, screening for infection is cost effective in pure financial terms[21,22].

Dynamic modelling undertaken for the CMO Expert Advisory Group for *C. trachomatis* indicated that screening would be cost effective[10]. However payment to healthcare professionals for undertaking initial screening tests was not included in the calculation. Further work on cost effectiveness is required. As more is understood about natural history and data are available from recent research projects, the probability estimates will need to be modified appropriately.

HOW SHOULD SCREENING BE UNDERTAKEN?

The CMO Expert Advisory Group on *C. trachomatis* concluded that screening and effective management of chlamydial infection would result in considerable health benefits. However evidence for the most cost effective approach to screening is lacking. There are many different facets of the initiatives in Scandinavia that produced a reduction in chlamydial infection.

The choice of opportunistic screening offered to known "high risk" groups was suggested as more appropriate than a register-based universal screening programme, with call and recall. The National Screening Committee in the UK supported piloting opportunistic screening in the Wirral and Portsmouth[23]. The final analysis should be available in 2001. The Health Technology Assessment Programme has also funded a large research project to address some of the outstanding questions with regard to mechanics of a screening programme.

Meanwhile there have been some professional and public educational initiatives albeit in a piece meal fashion. However, by engaging the media in its many forms, and with introduction of new guidelines on Sex and Relationship Education in schools, the general knowledge base of the population, and particularly the 'at risk' population, should improve. It is also important that the healthcare professionals have the necessary skills to support a screening programme. The Royal Colleges and Specialist Societies have started to work collaboratively to address the multi-disciplinary approach to management of genital chlamydial infection. With the uncontrolled epidemic in the UK at present, the reasons for offering widespread screening for *C. trachomatis* are compelling.

REFERENCES

1. Scholes D, Stergachis A, Heidrich FE, Andrilla H, Holmes KK, Stamm WE. (1996). Prevention of pelvic inflammatory disease by screening for cervical chlamydial infection. *NEJM* **334:** 1362–1366
2. Herrmann BF, Hohansson AB, Mardh P-A. (1991). A retrospective study of efforts to diagnose infections by *Chlamydia trachomatis* in a Swedish county. *Sex Trans Dis* **18:** 233–237.
3. Addis DG, Vaughn ML, Ludka D, Pfister J, Davis JP. (1993). Decreased prevalence of *Chlamydia trachomatis* infection associated with a selective screening programme in family planning clinics in Wisconsin. *Sex Trans Dis* **20:** 28–34.
4. Catchpole M, Pimenta J, Rogers P, Hopwood J, Randal S, Mallinson H, (2000). Opportunistic Screening for *Chlamydia trachomatis*; Methodology and preliminary results from a UK pilot study, Proceedings of the 4th Meeting of the European Society for Chlamydia Research 2000, p. 414.

5. Lamagni TL, Hughes G, Rogers PA, Paine T, Catchpole M. (1999). New cases seen at genitourinary medicine clinics: England 1998 *Commun Dis Rep CDR* S1–12.
6. Bevan CD, Johal BJ, Mumtaz G, Ridgway G, Siddle NC. (1995). Clinical, laparoscopic and microbiological findings in acute salpingitis: report on a United Kingdom cohort. *Br J Obstet Gynaecol* **102**: 407–14.
7. Buchan H, Vessey M, Goldacre M, Fairweather JTI. (1993). Morbidity following pelvic inflammatory disease. *Br J Obstet Gynaecol.* Jun; **100**(6): 558–62.
8. Page H, (1989). Estimation of the prevalence and incidence of infertility in a population: a pilot study. *Fertil-Steril.* Apr; **51**(4): 571–7.
9. Hull MG, Glazener CM, Kelly NJ, Conway DI, Foster PA, Hinton RA, Coulson C, Lambert PA, Watt EM, Desai KM. (1985). Population study of causes, treatment and outcome of infertility. *Br Med J Clin Res Ed.* Dec 14: **291**(6150): 1693–7.
10. Turner H, Townshend J: Modelling for Chlamydia Screening in: Chief Medical Officers Expert Advisory Group. Main Report of CMOs Expert Advisory Group on *Chlamydia trachomatis.* London: Department of Health, 1998. (Chapter 11)
11. Neuer A, Spandorfer S D, Giraldo P, Dieterle S, Rosenwax Z, Whitkin SS, (2000). The Role of Heat Shock Proteins in Reproduction, *Human Reproduction Update 2000;* **6**: 149–159.
12. Singh G, Blackwell A. (1994). Morbidity in male partners of women who have chlamydial infection before termination of pregnancy. *Lancet* **344**: 1438.
13. Blackwell Al, Thomas PD, Wareham K, Emery SJ. (1993). Health gains from screening for infection of the lower genital tract in women attending for termination of pregnancy. *Lancet* **342**: 206–209.
14. Farley TM, Rowe PJ, Rosenberg MJ, Chen J, Meirik O. (1992). Intrauterine devices and pelvic inflammatory disease: an international perspective. *Lancet* **339**: 785–788.
15. Ripa T. (1990). Epidemiologic control of genital *Chlamydia trachomatis* infections. *Scan J Infect Dis* (Suppl) **16**: 157–167.
16. Carder C, Robinson AJ, Broughton C, Stephenson JM, Ridgway GL. (1999). Evaluation of self-taken samples for the presence of genital *Chlamydia trachomatis* infection in women using the ligase chain reaction assay. *Int J STD & AIDS* **10**: 776–779.
17. Burstein GR, Gaydos CA, Diener-West M, Howell MR, Zenilman JM, Quinn TC. (1998). Incident *Chlamydia trachomatis* infections among inner-city adolescent females. *JAMA* **280**: 521–526.
18. Kjar HO, Dimcevski G, Hoff G, Olesen F, Ostergaard L. Recurrence of Urogenital *Chlamydia trachomatis* Infection Evaluated by Mailed Samples Obtained at Home; 24 weeks prospective follow-up study. *Sexually Transmitted Infections* (in print)
19. Washington AE, Browner WS, Korenbrot CC. (1987). Cost-effectiveness of combined treatment for endocervical gonorrhoea. Considering co-infection with *Chlamydia trachomatis. JAMA* **257**: 2056–60.
20. Washington AE, Johnson Re, Sanders LL Jr. (1987). *Chlamydia trachomatis* infections in the United States. What are they costing us? *JAMA* **257**: 2070–2.
21. Paavonen J, Puolakkainen M, Paukku M, Sintonen H, (1998). Cross Benefit Analysis of First Catch Urine, *Chlamydia trachomatis* screening programme. *Obstet Gynaecol* **92**: 292–8.
22. Genc M, Mardh A. (1996). A Cost Effectiveness Analysis of Screening and Treatment for *Chlamydia trachomatis* Infection in Asymptomatic Women. *Ann Intern Med* **124**: 1–7.
23. Pimenta, J, Catchpole, M, Grey M, Hopwood J, Randall S, (2000). Screening for Genital Chlamydial Infection, *Br Med J* **321**: 629–631.

CHAPTER 3

The Diagnosis of Chlamydia Trachomatis *Genital Infection*

E Owen Caul
The Public Health Laboratory, Bristol, UK

Alan J Herring
Genitourinary Infections Reference Laboratory, Bristol, UK

INTRODUCTION

In assessing diagnostic tests for *C. trachomatis* it is important to appreciate that various methods measure distinct targets which have different properties and are only loosely linked in terms of the amounts of target present in any given sample. Culture only detects viable chlamydial elementary bodies (EBs), the infectious form of Chlamydia. The enzyme-linked immunoassays (EIAs) detect chlamydial lipopolysaccharide (LPS) that is often found outside EBs in chlamydial inclusions and may be found in abundance in specimens with low numbers of mature EBs. Nucleic acid hybridization and amplification tests (NAHTs and NAATs) detect DNA and RNA and these differ in abundance with RNA in an approximately hundredfold excess. However, RNA is more labile than DNA which in turn is less stable than LPS. DNA and especially RNA are found in reticulate bodies which are present in clinical specimens. All of these considerations mean that only fresh clinical specimens are suitable for analytical comparisons whilst artificial, reconstituted specimens may bias the assessment.

SPECIMENS FOR DIAGNOSIS

There has been a significant change in recent years in the specimens used for the various assays. Historically, culture relied on cervical and urethral swabs (CSs and USs). These specimens are normally taken as part of a genital examination and, while appropriate for the genitourinary medicine clinic, may present difficulties in other healthcare settings due to the need for special equipment and time constraints. Cervical swabs need to be taken with great care and may cause discomfort and bleeding. Pooling the CS with a US increases detection rates since some women are infected only in the urethra but this adds to the discomfort. Male urethral swabs for chlamydial diagnosis require deep insertion which many patients find painful. For these reasons, inadequately taken swab specimens have been a widely reported problem.

More recently the utility of non-invasive specimens has become established. The initial report showed that male first catch urine (FCU) is a suitable alternative specimen when tested by amplified EIA[1]. Subsequently, female FCU was found to be an adequate specimen for the NAATs[2]. While this was a considerable advance, the use of FCUs requires centrifugation and this extra step adds considerably to laboratory processing time. Recently, many groups have found that vulvo/vaginal swabs (VVSs) give better sensitivity than urine and avoid the need to centrifuge[3]. Preliminary measurements of the amount of chlamydial DNA in female FCUs and vulvo/vaginal swabs also indicate that swabs provide fewer specimens with very low DNA values[4] although, interestingly, for males the distribution of DNA is similar for US and FCU specimens. However, the acceptability of VVSs to women may be less than that of a urine specimen.

This move to non-invasive specimens has had a major impact on the design of screening programmes since specimens can now be taken easily in a range of healthcare settings or even in the home. Unfortunately, the degree to which this advance can be exploited is limited to some extent by specimen stability. FCUs left at ambient temperature show a reduced sensitivity when assayed by NAATs[5] and the manufacturers recommend a cold chain for such specimens. The addition of boric acid can aid stability of urine[3]. Initial data suggest the stability of VVSs is better but more investigation is required. In contrast, the LPS detected by EIAs is thermostable and transport stability is not a problem.

As well as the genital tract, *C. trachomatis* also infects the eye and rectal mucosa. Swabs from the conjuctiva are suitable specimens for all diagnostic methods but rectal swabs are not appropriate for EIA tests due to the high frequency of false positives.

DESCRIPTION OF THE TESTS

Culture
In terms of routine diagnosis, culture has no role in most modern laboratories.

Its sole function outside research is for the investigation of sexual abuse cases. It is considered to be 100% specific and is the only test currently recognised in medico-legal cases. It is likely that this situation will have to change since the lack of local culture facilities is becoming a limiting factor in medico-legal investigations.

Direct Immunofluorescent Assays
In direct immunofluorescent assays (DIF) polyclonal or monoclonal antibodies with a fluorescent label are used to detect infected cells in smears made from a variety of specimens. The antibodies react with either genus-specific epitopes (LPS) or species-specific epitopes on the major outer membrane protein (MOMP). The anti-MOMP reagents stain EBs and results are much easier to interpret since the size and morphology of the EB is distinctive. These reagents are particularly suitable for the confirmation of EIAs or NAATs. Genus specific anti-LPS antibodies react with EBs, reticulate bodies (RBs) and free LPS and this last component tends to give high background fluorescence. This means they are best used for detecting chlamydial inclusions, as in confirming positive cell cultures or examining eye swabs in cases of chlamydial conjuctivitis. Cross reactions with other bacteria are not a problem as morphological criteria can be used in their differentiation.

The quality of the smears is of paramount importance to achieving high sensitivities with these reagents. Following the preparation of the smear (CS, US, rectal or conjuctival) the slide is fixed in acetone or methanol prior to staining with antibody reagent. An important advantage of DIF is that it is the only method that allows the quality of the specimen to be assessed during diagnosis.

Conventional Enzyme-linked Immunoassays (EIAs)
A large number of different EIAs are available and they all detect chlamydial LPS through an antigen capture method. The monoclonal or polyclonal antibodies used for capture recognise Chlamydia-specific epitopes in the oligosaccharide core of the LPS. The assays detect captured LPS complexes using a conventional enzyme-labelled antibody which produces a signal through a colour or chemiluminescence generating substrate.

Amplified Enzyme-linked Immunoassays
In this format, antigen is captured normally but signal generation is amplified by two mechanisms. First, the antibody is conjugated with a linker such that

each antibody molecule carries several enzyme molecules. Second, an additional enzyme system is added to the reaction which serves to increase the colour producing reaction by substrate regeneration. However, the significant differences in the sensitivities of EIA's can be attributed not only to the assay design but also to the avidity of the particular antibody used in the assay.

Confirmation of Enzyme-linked Immunoassays
Because some bacteria can bind immunoglobulins they can produce false colour in EIAs and we have found recently that lubricant preparations such as 'KY gel' can also interfere with amplified EIA. It is therefore essential to confirm EIA positives with another test to achieve a high specificity. Confirmation can be achieved by a blocking reaction with an unlabelled second antibody, by DIF or by a NAAT. However, many laboratories now extend their confirmation to include specimens in the 'negative' grey-zone below the manufacturer's cut-off value to maximize sensitivity. These grey-zone specimens cannot be confirmed by a blocking assay but many are positive with DIF or a NAAT. The latter is our favoured methodology because DIF requires extensive experience and is unsuitable for high throughputs[6].

Automation of Enzyme-linked Immunoassays
EIAs can be utilised in manual, semi-automated or completely automated mode. Laboratory workers need to be aware that automated plate washing lines can become contaminated with microorganisms with antibody binding properties that can result in high background noise. All equipment should be thoroughly cleansed on a regular basis prior to use for EIA assays. The use of automation gives EIA a throughput far greater than that currently achievable by NAATs.

Nucleic Acid Hybridization Tests
The first commercial nucleic acid-based test was the 'Genprobe PACE' system (Genprobe Inc., San Diego, CA) which detects *C. trachomatis*-specific sequences in ribosomal RNA (rRNA) using an acridinium ester-labelled hybridization probe. Hybrids are detected by magnetic bead capture and reading the chemiluminescent signal from the probe. An unlabelled 'blocking' probe can be used for confirmation in a manner analogous to the blocking antibody in EIA.

Recently, another hybridization test has appeared – the Digene Hybrid Capture assay (Digene, Beltsville, MD) which uses an unlabelled RNA probe complementary to 5% of the *C. trachomatis* genome. After lysis and hybridization in solution, the hybrids are captured using an antibody against RNA/DNA hybrids and are detected using the same antibody conjugated with alkaline phosphatase in conjunction with a chemiluminescent substrate.

Nucleic Acid Amplification Tests (NAATs)

All these assays rely for their specificity on the hybridization reactions of their primers and for their sensitivity on the activity of various polymerases and other modifying enzymes that synthesize the amplified target. The original amplification method was the polymerase chain reaction (PCR). The PCR and the ligase chain reaction (LCR), both require heat denaturation in a 'thermocycler' to separate DNA strands for the next round of reactions, while for Transcript Mediated Amplification (TMA) and Strand Displacement Amplification (SDA) the reaction occurs at a constant temperature.

Polymerase Chain Reaction

The first, standardised, commercial *C. trachomatis* PCR kit, 'Amplicor CT', was launched by Roche Diagnostics Inc. (Pleasanton, CA, USA). This is a manual assay that can accommodate all specimen types. DNA is released from the specimen with lysis buffer, followed by addition of a 'master mix' containing the labeled primers, polymerase, deoxynucleotides and PCR reaction buffer and then thermocycling. Product is detected by capture using hybridization probes immobilised onto the wells of a microtitre plate. Biotin label incorporated into the primers is detected with peroxidase-labelled strepavidin in a colourimetric reaction.

The manual kit was followed by an automated version called the Roche 'Cobas Amplicor CT'. The machine performs essentially the same steps as the manual assay with the exception that hybrid capture was achieved with oligonucleotide probes immobilised onto magnetic beads rather than microtitre plate wells.

Two important additions are now incorporated into the Roche PCR assays. To counter the threat of amplicon contamination, an enzyme system is used which specifically digests amplicon but not target DNA. Optionally, an internal control sequence which uses a separate set of primers can be added. Failure of this sequence to amplify indicates the presence of inhibitors of the amplification reaction in the clinical sample.

Ligase Chain Reaction

In the LCR reaction four primers are positioned very closely on the same DNA target separated by a gap of a few nucleotides. In addition to Taq polymerase, the reaction incorporates a thermostable ligase and primers are complementary to both DNA target strands. Product is thus generated by both strands at once and consists of continuous, ligated DNA molecule containing two primer sequences. The primers incorporate two labels, one of which is used for capture and the other for detection. Amplicons are trapped on microparticles, washed by filtration and detected using an alkaline phosphatase-labelled antibody and a fluorescence producing substrate. LCR assays are available only in the automated form ('LCx', Abbott Diagnostics, IL, USA) and require a dedicated thermocycler and a detection module

Both PCR and LCR target the cryptic plasmid of *C. trachomatis* which is present at 4-10 copies per copy of genomic DNA.

Transcript Mediated Amplification
The Genprobe 'Amplified CT' assay targets rRNA and begins by the hybridization of a DNA primer which has at its 5' end a phage RNA polymerase promoter sequence. The primer targets a Chlamydia-specific sequence in 16S rRNA. This primer is then extended by reverse transcriptase and the RNA complement is removed by RNase H activity. A second primer then binds to the end of this DNA and is extended backwards to give a double stranded DNA template which can be transcribed by a phage polymerase to give multiple transcripts, some of which are themselves converted into templates. The RNA product is detected using an acridinium-labelled probe as in the PACE assay (see above). The TMA assay was offered initially as a manual system but recently the assay has also been developed to run on the 'Vidas' platform (Pasteur Merieux).

Strand Displacement Amplification (SDA)
The Becton Dickinson (Maryland, USA) 'Probetec ET' relies on the property of DNA polymerase to synthesize a new strand on the 3' side of a nick in the backbone of DNA while displacing the existing strand from the duplex. This nick is introduced by a restriction endonuclease which only cleaves one strand because the other strand has incorporated αS substituted dCTP during a complex set of template-producing 'priming' reactions. These reactions involve 4 primers which once again target a sequence in the cryptic plasmid. An initial lysis/denaturation step at 100°C is required, followed by priming at 75°C and amplification at 52°C.

As well as the novel amplification chemistry, the Probetec test is the first to incorporate closed tube detection of amplicon with a fluorescent probe. There are several different designs of such probes but all work by modifying the fluorescence output of the primary fluorochrome by changing its location relative to a quenching or enhancing secondary fluorochrome. In the Probetec system, emission from a fluorescein molecule is quenched by a proximal rhodamine. When the probe binds to the amplicon the two molecules are separated and emitted light escapes. The advantages of this technique are that it allows measurement in real time without the necessity to open the tube and risk contamination.

THE RELATIVE MERITS OF THE ASSAYS

The literature on *C. trachomatis* assays needs considerable care in interpretation. Many modern assays exceed the sensitivity of culture which was originally considered the 'gold standard'. This has led to a difficult situation in which many researchers have used 'discrepant analysis' in which extra tests are performed only on those specimens giving an anomalous result. This has led to an acrimonious and long running argument with the statisticians regarding the calculation of sensitivities and specificities. A discussion of this problem was recently published by McAdam[7]. Lack of a gold standard means that comparisons of sensitivities and specificities between studies are fraught with difficulties. Many studies confirm that there is no single test/specimen combination that will detect all infected individuals.

Several considerations bear on the decision of which assay to use but undoubtedly the most important are sensitivity and specificity, cost and required throughput. Specificity is not a particular problem since all the common assays have specificities in the high 90% range when used properly although for the EIAs this means in conjunction with a confirmatory test. However, NAATs have the special problem that their normally high specificity can be undermined by contamination giving false positives. Repeat testing is only a partial answer as the residual specimen may be contaminated[8]. Neither does failure to repeat necessarily indicate contamination since the ability of the assays to detect very low numbers of molecules leads to irreproducibility simply because of random distribution of the target. Routine statistical analyses of the level and pattern of occurrence of positive specimens as described by Shapiro[9] are a sensible precaution and should be performed before results are reported. Strict adherence to cleaning and maintenance protocols for automated platforms is also essential to avoid false positives.

There is no doubt that the NAATs are the most sensitive assays with typical values around or exceeding 90%. All the current NAATs have their sensitivity limited by inhibition which is reported to affect between 2.6% and 7.5% of all urine specimens[10]. Currently, only the Roche PCR and the BD Probetec have internal controls to detect this problem. The actual inhibitors vary for each assay but freezing or dilution usually overcomes the inhibitory effect[10]. Detailed 'head to head' comparisons of all the NAATs have not been performed and most experienced workers are inclined to view them all as highly sensitive and specific. The decision of which NAAT to use is more likely to be guided by considerations of cost, space requirements and work practices. The costs of NAATs can vary considerably with volume purchased and other considerations but are high relative to other assays.

The choice of test for the majority of laboratories has been EIA. This has been because of the large cost differential between EIA and NAATs. The cheapest NAAT is at present 4 times as expensive as a typical EIA and, until recently, this ratio was even greater. The literature is a poor guide to their relative performance as reported sensitivities of EIAs relative to NAATs vary from 0% to nearly 100%! Many of the most unfavourable comparisons in the literature used first generation, conventional EIAs.

A recent paper from Japan reported equivalent sensitivities for the Dako 'PCE' amplified EIA (Dako Diagnostics Ltd., Cambridgeshire, UK) and the Roche PCR for both CSs and VVSs[11]. This study was small and used a high prevalence population but very recently the result for CSs has been confirmed by a Canadian group sampling a population with only 4% prevalence[12]. They found an amplified EIA sensitivity relative to LCR of 90%. We are aware of three independent, unpublished studies that support this value for CSs. Thus, contrary to many reports, we believe that modern amplified EIA tests can provide an acceptable level of performance when used on CSs.

However, it is clear that in the future many specimens will be non-invasive. Recently, we have performed a much larger amplified EIA/PCR comparison on VVSs. We used The Dako PCE with DIF confirmation including grey-zone specimens and found a sensitivity of 90% relative to PCR. Since we also found performance with male urine is highly satisfactory, we believe that EIAs may have a role in screening programmes, especially in situations in which cost is a dominant factor.

The role of NAHTs, which are intermediate in price between EIA and NAAT, remains unclear. The Genprobe PACE assay is less sensitive than NAATs. It has been widely used in the USA largely because it was the first

Table 1. Overview of *C. trachomatis* diagnostic assays

Test	Transport	Cost	Advantages	Disadvantages
Culture	Must reach lab. in 24hrs	High, especially labour costs	Only test for medico legal work	Needs skilled technicians
Conventional EIA	No cold chain	Low	Simple, high throughput	Sensitivities vary greatly, needs confirmation
Amplified EIA	No cold chain	Low	Simple, high throughput, good sensitivity and specificity	Needs confirmation
Direct Immuno-Fluorescence	No cold chain	Low (high labour costs)	Good for confirmation of other tests and research	Quality of results depend on experience of technician. Throughput very limited
NAATS	Cold chain required	High kit and labour costs	Highest sensitivity and specificity	Needs a lot of lab space. Contamination is a constant threat

system to provide a parallel test for *Neisseria gonorrhoeae*. If a test for gonorrhoea is required, all the above NAATs also have this feature. Avoiding the need for a gonococcus culture changes the relative economics of the tests. In this review, we have concentrated on the situation in which the gonococcus prevalence is low. The Digene assay can also detect gonococcus. It is labour intensive in its current form but is reported to perform well in comparison to PCR[13] and has recently been automated.

National screening programmes will demand high throughputs and this inevitably means automation. The automation of EIAs is similar to that for serology, a variety of robots are available and give very high throughputs.

The complete automation of NAATs currently presents a formidable problem. While not presently a commercially available system, successful automation of the Roche Amplicor assay has been achieved in a major

American private diagnostic laboratory and will ultimately achieve throughputs of around 2000 wells per day which can be attributed to Chlamydia, gonococcus or internal control as desired. The Genprobe 'Amplified *C. trachomatis*' will currently run on the Vidas automation. Genprobe have also announced the next generation of their test ('Tigris-Aptima') which is a fully automated system purifying target from specimens by hybrid capture and using it in an improved TMA assay system. The system will allow parallel testing for gonococcus, have considerably enhanced throughput and, since it purifies target, should eliminate inhibition. Several robots have been released recently which isolate nucleic acid for research tests but, while currently in use for blood screening, they have not yet been applied to chlamydial diagnosis. Becton Dickinson is also known to be producing an automated system to prepare samples for the 'Probetec' assay.

All these systems are aimed squarely at large scale screening programmes and their performance and reliability will take time to assess. In terms of current manual systems, the BD Probetec and the Genprobe amplified *C. trachomatis* both allow more specimens to be processed in a day per diagnostic set up. High throughput with the LCx or Cobas PCR requires multiple machines that are expensive and space consuming.

The relative strengths of the various methods are summarised in **Table 1**.

FUTURE DEVELOPMENTS

Chlamydia diagnosis remains a highly competitive commercial area that attracts considerable effort. We have avoided the subject of near patient testing in this review because the current generation of tests is not yet sensitive enough to be truly useful. There is clearly a need for a sensitive, low cost screening assay, especially in the developing world, as witnessed by the offer of a considerable prize by the Rockefeller Foundation and substantial support by the Wellcome Foundation and WHO. Driven mostly by the threat of bio-terrorism, research into novel, ultra-sensitive detection systems is moving very rapidly. Recent advances may well mean that antigen or nucleic acid detection in novel electronic devices or even a totally automated form of DIF by an image analysis robot will provide very rapid diagnosis in the future.

REFERENCES

1. Caul EO, Paul ID, Milne J, Crowley T, (1988). Non-invasive sampling method for detecting *Chlamydia trachomatis*. *Lancet* **I**:1246-47.

2. Lee HH, Chernesky MA, Schachter, J. *et al.* (1995). Diagnosis of *Chlamydia trachomatis* genitourinary infection in women by ligase chain reaction of urine. *Lancet 345* **8444:** 213–216.
3. Carder C, Robinson AJ, Broughton C *et al.* (1999). Evaluation of self-taken samples for the presence of genital *Chlamydia trachomatis* infection in women using the ligase chain reaction assay.
4. Michel CE, Hagley M, Carne C. *et al.* (2000). Quantitation of *Chlamydia trachomatis* load at multiple genitorinary sites: implication for screening strategy. In 'Proceedings of the 4th meeting of the European Society for Chlamydia research. Ed. Saikku, P. Univesitas Helsingiensis.
5. Caul EO, Horner PJ, Leece J *et al.* (1997). Population-based screening programmes for *Chlamydia trachomatis*. *Lancet* **349:**1070–71.
6. Dean D, Ferrero D and McCarthy M. (1998). Comparison of performance and cost-effectiveness of direct fluorescent-antibody, ligase chain reaction and PCR assays for verification of chlamydial enzyme immunoassays results for populations with low to moderate prevalence of *Chlamydia trachomatis* infection. *J Clin Microbiol* **36:** 94–99.
7. McAdam AJ. (2000). Discrepant analysis: how can we test a test. *J Clin Microbiol* **38:** 2027–2029.
8. Gronowski AM, Copper S, Baorto D. *et al.* (2000). Reproducibility problems with the Abbott LCx assay for *Chlamydia trachomatis* and *Neisseria gonorrhoeae*. *J Clin Microbiol* **38:** 2416–8.
9. Shapiro DS. (1999) Quality contol in nucleic acid amplification methods: Use of elementary probability theory. *J Clin Microbiol* **37:** 848–851.
10. Mahony JB, Chong S, Jang D. *et al.* (1998). Urine specimens from pregnant and non-pregnant women inhibitory to amplification of *Chlamydia trachomatis* nucleic acic by PCR, ligase chain reaction and transcript-mediated amplication: identification of urinary substances associated with inhibition and removal of inhibitory activity. *J Clin Microbiol* **36:** 3122–3126
11. Tanaka M, Nakayama H, Yoshida H. *et al.* (1998). Detection of *Chlamydia trachomatis* in vaginal specimens from female commercial sex workers using a new improved enzyme immunoassay. *Sex Transm Inf* **74:** 435–438.
12. Chernesky MA, Jang D, Copes D. *et al.* (2000). Use of an enzme amplified immunoassay (IDEIA PCE) and LCR to detect *Chlamydia trachomatis* in cervical swabs. In 'Proceedings of the 4th meeting of the European Society for Chlamydia research. Ed. Saikku, P. Univesitas Helsingiensis.
13. Girdiner JL, Cullen AP, Salama TG. *et al.* (1999). Evaluation of the Digene Hybrid Capture II CT-ID test for detection of *Chlamydia trachomatis* in endocervical specimens. *J Clin Microbiol* **37:** 1579–1581.

CHAPTER 4

Human genital infections with Chlamydia Trachomatis – *is there a role for serology?*

Timothy R Moss
Genito-Urinary Medicine, Doncaster Royal Infirmary

Sohrab Darougar
University of London, UK

INTRODUCTION

The worldwide prevalence and incidence of *Chlamydia trachomatis* genital infection (CTGI) is estimated to be 700 million and 90 million respectively. In the USA and Western Europe, the number of new cases of CTGI is estimated to exceed (respectively) 4 and 5.5 million per annum. The true prevalence and incidence of CTGI may be 2 to 3 times higher if cases of chronic CTGI with mild symptoms and asymptomatic cases were included.

Several authors have acknowledged the problem of the large number of asymptomatic cases of human genital chlamydial infection (50-80%) in which no clinical presentation is made,[1] or where there are symptoms and signs which are generally mild and indistinguishable from those of other sexually transmitted diseases (STDs).

Indeed, it may be appropriate to regard the majority of chlamydial genital tract infections in both men and women as a potentially chronic disease with an insidious onset.

In men and women with CTGI spontaneous recovery may occur in a small number of cases.

Frequently CTGIs may persist for months or years causing serious complications in both sexes,[2] especially females. Chronic/long term infection may be associated with the shedding of a very low numbers of infectious elementary bodies, or intermittent shedding. In these patients the sensitivity of conventional antigen detection tests is low. Nucleic Acid amplification assays such as Polymerase chain reaction (PCR) and Ligase chain reaction (LCR) may increase positivity rates by up to 30%.

Immunological responses in human chlamydial diseases vary. In the case of *C. trachomatis* serovars A, B, B & C (trachoma) immunological responses appear to be predominantly cellular.

This contrasts with the serovars L1, 2 and 3 of lymphogranuloma venereum (LGV) where cellular responses deal promptly with the initial skin lesion; but the disseminated lymph node involvement, and other complications (such as polyarthritis) prompt rising antibody titres detectable by the LGV complement fixation test. Exposure to the genitourinary serovars (D-K) results in a distinct cellular response. Humoral responses have received increasing attention in recent years.

In this chapter it is intended to discuss the possibility that chlamydial serological responses may offer a useful adjunct to the diagnosis and understanding of genito-urinary chlamydial infections and their complications.

Serological responses will be considered within the context of serial observations, in combination with antigen detection systems, and within the context of the clinical complexity, extent, and duration of the disease process.

DIAGNOSIS

The diagnosis of genital chlamydial infection relies entirely on laboratory tests. Methods of diagnosis based on isolation of the organism, detecting its infectious elementary bodies using mononuclear antibodies or detecting its components by enzyme immunoassay (EIA) are sensitive during the acute phase of the infection. They are, however, of low sensitivity in cases of chronic or repeated chlamydial infections. There is debate as to whether these tests are cost effective in low risk populations.[3]

Although high rates of infection were identified in asymptomatic teenage women, Clay[4] emphasised that opportunistic screening and treatment will fail to reduce the prevalence of Chlamydia without co-ordinated contact tracing and follow-up. The proposed UK Nationwide screening model sees this process as essential.[5] The range and application of antigen detection in diagnosis is covered by Dr Caul and Dr Herring (Chapter 3).

Reference is made to the highly competitive effort currently in progress to produce a sensitive, low cost screening assay via greater sophistication of antigen detection.

The further development and application of serological tests may also be regarded as a valid and urgent priority. This is of particular importance with regard to recurrent, latent, subacute and chronic disease.

THE PRESENT STATUS OF CHLAMYDIA SEROLOGY

False positive results can occur in Chlamydia serology; for example with L2 based tests due to cross reactivity to antibodies produced to *C. pneumoniae* which is widely prevalent in Europe and the USA. This has led to a widespread belief that there is little place for Chlamydia serology in the diagnosis of human genital infections.

A variety of serological tests including complement-fixation, agglutination, haemagglutination, immunodiffusion, haemolysis in gel and radioimmune precipitation tests have been used in the past. These tests detect group-specific antibodies and have a very low sensitivity and specificity for detecting chlamydial antibodies. The methods commonly used today are complement fixation, indirect immunofluorescence (IFT), enzyme immunoassay (EIA) and microimmunofluorescence (MIF) tests.

In IFT or EIA, infected cells with one CT serotype, purified elementary bodies of a CT serotype or a pool of CT serotypes D to K are used as a single antigen. These tests detect group-specific chlamydial antibodies and cannot differentiate between antibody responses to CTDK, *C. pneumoniae* and *C. psittaci*. In contrast the MIF test detects and separates antibodies to CT from those to non-genital Chlamydia species including *C. pneumoniae* and *C. psittaci*. The original MIF test is a complex technology requiring deposition of microdots of all chlamydial serotype antigens individually and a complicated method of reading, recording and analysis of results. Subsequently, simplified versions of MIF were developed to detect type-specific antibodies to Chlamydia species.

In our laboratory we used a modified MIF test developed by Treharne *et al.*[6] In summary the test consists of the following: samples of blood are collected by venepuncture. The sera can be tested immediately or stored at +4°C for testing after a few days or stored at −20°C for a longer period.

The antigens consist of panels of microdots containing egg grown purified elementary bodies of Chlamydia serovars. Each panel contains four antigen microdots representing:

1) a pool of *C. trachomatis* serovars D to K,
2) single *C. psittaci* agent, IOL 395 isolated in the virus laboratory, Institute

of Ophthalmology, London, from the eyes of a human with acute conjunctivitis. This organism cross-reacts with reference sera against other *C. psittaci* strains including 33L, isolated from a case of lymphogranuloma venereum, A22/18, a ewe abortion agent, and a pigeon chlamydial agent,

3) a single *C. pneumoniae agent* IOL 207, isolated from the eye of a child with clinical signs of trachoma in Iran. IOL-207 is serologically similar to TW183, a *C. pneumoniae* strain isolated from the eye of a patient in Taiwan,

4) a negative control using uninfected yolk sacs prepared the same way as infected yolk sacs.

Serum specimens are tested for the presence of IgG at a starting dilution of 1/16 and IgM at a starting dilution of 1/8 using an indirect immuno-fluorescence staining technique. The presence of specific antibodies to CTDK only or cross-reactive against 2 or 3 species, with the highest level against CTDK are considered to identify a CTDK response.

Thomas *et al* [7] (2000) used the Micro Immuno Fluorescence technique to assess the significance of positive serology in fallopian tube disease. They reported a marked association between level of titre and the likelihood of tubal damage.

Laparoscopy has been regarded as the Gold Standard diagnostic method for pelvic inflammatory disease but this affords limited information regarding endo tubal morphology. In particular, no insight is afforded with regard to cilial function and physiology. With antigen tests of cervical and tubal material proving negative in some cases; the need for further development in serological testing is emphasised.

Thomas therefore argued that by using *C. trachomatis* antibody testing more widely it may be possible to reduce the number of laparoscopies performed, and that MIF Chlamydia serology should become an integral part of infertility investigation.

The potential value of using both McCoy cell culture systems in isolating *C. trachomatis* and serological tests for Chlamydia was argued as early as in 1987.[8] It was suggested that the use of Micro Immuno Fluorescent Chlamydia serology may be a useful adjunct to tests for antigen from the endocervix and fallopian tubes. One early conclusion was that the addition of species specific Chlamydia serology to the routine investigation of women presenting with pelvic inflammatory disease undoubtedly aids the identification of those infected with *C. trachomatis*. Furthermore, if recurrences of pelvic infection are to be minimised, these women require prolonged tetracycline or erythromycin therapy as well as investigation and treatment of their sexual partner(s).

Examples of such cases will be discussed later in this chapter.

A preceding local study (1986)[9] supported this concept. The untreated, asymptomatic male partner of a woman with PID is an important aetiological factor in the recurrent nature of this disease.

Seventy-one women were reviewed who had a clinical diagnosis of acute pelvic inflammatory disease (PID). 40.8% of women with acute PID had evidence of chlamydial infection using a combination of McCoy cell culture/antigen detection and MIF serology. All of these women were counselled and advised to ask their current sexual partner/partners to attend the GU clinic for investigation. This process was patient led, supported by counselling from health advisers and/or ward based nursing staff.

Forty-five male partners were seen and screened for genital tract infection by conventional methods. Of the 45 male partners investigated >2 out of 3 had recoverable Chlamydia in their anterior urethra. It was of particular interest to find that Chlamydia was isolated from some men whose female partners were culture negative but D-K IgG positive. These men were frequently asymptomatic carriers.

At this time, chlamydial pelvic inflammatory disease in Doncaster appeared to be five times more common than gonococcal PID. Combined infections were frequent. Some of these cases may, represent "*quiescent chlamydial infection*". Latent chlamydial infection with serovars D-K may (like *C. pneumoniae*) be unmasked by another infection. Serology may support this interpretation.

It was concluded that unless regular male consorts are fully investigated; and additional consorts are also traced, we cannot anticipate containment of chlamydial genital infection in communities.

The role of serology was subjected to further study by the same group and reported in 1993.[10]

Over 7000 cases attending the Genito Urinary Medicine (GU) clinic in Doncaster between May 1983 and May 1990 were assessed serologically using the modified Micro Immuno Fluorescent serology (MIF) test[10] (described above).

This study showed that antibodies to *C. pneumoniae* and *C. psittaci* accounted for up to 50% of all Chlamydia IgG positive cases. Infections with *C. pneumoniae* are universally widespread, and have been demonstrated serologically in up to 50% of the adult population in Europe and the United States.

The demonstration that IgG responses to *C. pneumoniae* and *C. psittaci* (i.e. non-genital pathogens) may account for up to half of all Chlamydia sero-positive cases attending GU clinics is important. This explains why less specific Chlamydia blood tests have not been found to be helpful, and why there has been little advocacy for the use of Chlamydia serology in clinical practice.

It is clearly necessary to recommend that serological tests which can differentiate antibodies to genito-urinary *C. trachomatis* serovars D-K (CTDK) from those to *C. pneumoniae* and *C. psittaci* should be the focus of further sero epidemiological studies.

Although there is a degree of cross reactivity in the MIF test system referred to, it appears possible to accurately identify D-K responses in most cases.

The accuracy of interpretation is believed to be enhanced by considering the IgG sero status within the clinical context; and preferably against the background of past and present antigen detection results and MIF species specific serology in both the presenting patient and in the sexual partner(s).

Clinical practice over some 20 years has allowed a very large, day to day experience of managing diagnostically discordant couples. The detection of one partner who is antigen positive and the other antigen negative but D-K IgG sero positive calls for the exclusion of complications in both. This may influence treatment considerations and long term follow-up.

Subsequently some 200 Chlamydia positive female patients were studied[11]. Infection was found in the same proportion of male partners. This work compared and contrasted McCoy cell culture with sero diagnosis; and also reviewed clinical diagnosis.

It was shown that in contacts of patients with genital chlamydial infection neither cell culture diagnosis, nor serotype specific serology testing (or clinical diagnosis) alone achieved the levels of sensitivity and specificity required for identifying current infection. It was proposed that selective application of both diagnostic modalities (preferably using PCR or LCR for antigen detection) may offer substantial improvement.

To repeat this study with a larger, prospective analysis would be of compelling interest. Clinical assessment should be more comprehensive. Clinical categorisation should distinguish symptomatic from latent/ asymptomatic/'carrier' cases. Evidence of disseminated male chlamydial disease should be sought such as prostatitis and sexually acquired reactive arthrosis (SARA) as well as complications in females.

There remains wide acceptance that improved antigen detection alone is not wholly satisfactory. It may in part be 'site dependent'. Kinghorn (personal communication) observed:- "It is well established that endo-cervical cultures for *C. trachomatis* may be negative in patients with active tubal infection:- (i.e. Chlamydia antigen positive – proven by laparoscopically obtained tubal specimens.)"

When species specific Chlamydia serology was combined with more modern antigen detection systems a marked increase in the sensitivity of diagnosis was achieved. This combined approach facilitates the identification and treatment of more cases of infectious genital chlamydial disease in populations – which minimises the very serious risk of female patients being subjected to multiple re-exposure to the pathogen from both exogenous and endogenous sources. There is subsequently a decreased risk in these women of 'amplified tissue damage' not only via a reduction of multiple episodes of exposure to D-K *C. trachomatis* in their genital tract, but also, by limiting or avoiding additional mucosal damage via the hypersensitivity response to the highly immunogenic heat shock protein (HSP60)[12] (or other inappropriate host mediated inflammatory responses) which are considered important in the pathogenesis of fallopian tube destruction by this organism. The fact that late, disseminated chlamydial genital infection in women is chronic, crippling and largely incurable provides another reason for improved serological diagnosis.

Chronic chlamydial infection almost invariably produces a scarring process. The pathogenesis of this scarring is unknown in detail despite the correlation with antibodies to certain epitopes on chlamydial heat shock proteins. A greater understanding of the patho-physiology of this scarring process may allow application of/development of drugs that would limit this process. For example Morton and Kinghorn advocated the use of proteolytics within this context. [13]

In 1991[14] Taylor Robinson stated: "the role of serology in diagnosis continues to be a contentious issue" He recommended caution because high titres do not always correlate with the detection of Chlamydia. It is well recognised that in late chlamydial disease, diagnosed serologically, negative antigen tests are most frequent. The use of a range of modalities of investigation, including the most recent developments in antigen detection, in combination with serology:- (and ideally, in conjunction with antigen detection and serology in the sexual partner) – may identify female cases justifying therapeutic intervention.

The complexities of GU chlamydial disease surely merit a greater effort to clarify the role of serology in diagnosis.

At a time when pilot studies of antigen screening for genital tract chlamydial disease have commenced, the wider application of serology could enhance our awareness of the prevalence of exposure to this group of pathogens in selected populations.

Rank[15] 1999, suggests that we are now on the threshold of understanding how the basic intracellular molecular interactions of the host cell and the organism may determine the nature of the immune response. It is possible that the interactions that Chlamydiae establish within the host cell may actually pre-determine the immune mechanisms (cellular and humoral), which the host may use to limit the infection. Brunham[16] discusses human immunity in the same text and offers a personal view of chlamydial immunity and immuno-pathology. It is suggested that the host facilitates persistent chlamydial infection via a failure to suppress growth at the epithelial cell level. This is due to an induced absence of protective host responses.

Chlamydiae are variably susceptible to inactivation by cellular and humoral defences. High serum antibody to GU Chlamydiae suggests persistent infection (see case 2), but the dilemma remains:- How do some organisms survive such defences to initiate and sustain recurrent episodes of infection? Whilst this question remains unanswered, and of fundamental importance, plausible hypotheses are beginning to emerge.[13]

Morton[17] has proposed three (theoretical) types of male carrier status:

1. Urethral carriers.
2. Prostatic carriers.
3. Lymph gland or splenic carriers.
   (Types 2 and 3 may of course present as Type 1)

Positive serology may help identify such carrier states. Treatment of these cases, and their long term serological follow-up alongside treated diseased patients might prove enlightening in terms of understanding residual infection and persistence/latency.

In busy Genito Urinary Medicine Departments the emphasis is on case finding and management of more acute disease. There is a further concern however:- is it possible to detect latent, or asymptomatic active disease by extended clinical surveillance and serological monitoring?

Whilst serodiagnosis of exposure to D-K serovars of *C. trachomatis* may contribute to the identification of 'latent' disease; this concept remains the most challenging in terms of clinical and laboratory diagnosis. Just as the diagnosis of late latent syphilis could only be made after exclusion of neurological or cardiovascular disease activity; so latent chlamydial infection demands at least exclusion of prostatitis in men, SARA in men and women and pelvic disease in women.

With existing serological tests it should be possible to establish a base line in terms of D-K IgG titres and to monitor changing titres against time in the long term surveillance of early disease recurrences and exacerbations of PID and Reiter's Syndrome/SARA :- especially in HLA A31 and B27 positive cases.

The presence of type specific antibodies to CTDK suggests that the patient has been exposed to the organism at some time. The natural history of CTGI would support the concept that a number of these patients will have a *current* infection. A judicious application of antimicrobial therapy for these patients *may* have potential benefits.

Work in Scandinavia and United States has demonstrated that the prevention of Pelvic Inflammatory Disease is achievable by actively screening and treating chlamydial cervical infection. The observation that PID may be present in the absence of detectable antigen in the cervix supports the view that species specific serology may improve the efficacy of this type of screening programme. A pilot study is indicated.

CASE REPORTS

Chlamydia and *in vitro* fertilisation embryo replacement (IVF/ER) and tubal infertility

Sero-epidemiological studies in patients undergoing IVF/ER further define the avoidable morbidity of female chlamydial infection in the upper genital tract.[18,19,20]

Chlamydial damage to the epithelial cilia within the fallopian tubes occurs early in both overt and covert pelvic inflammatory disease. Subsequent delay in transfer of the fertilised ovum through the tubal canal predisposes to ectopic gestation.

In women receiving IVF/ER with known tubal disease the serological evidence of exposure to Chlamydia D-K was, as expected, much higher than in those with non tubal causes for their infertility. (57% versus 13%)[20]

Of those women with history of both tubal disease and ectopic pregnancy, 69% had serological evidence of previous exposure to D-K serovars of *C. trachomatis.*

Case 1

It is believed that the first report of a possible relationship between previous exposure to *Chlamydia trachomatis* and failure of IVF/ER was reported by Moss and Steptoe.[21]

This was a case report where chlamydial infection in both husband and wife may have contributed to the loss of an implanted ovum on two occasions following *in vitro* fertilisation.

Extended antichlamydial therapy to both partners was followed by a successful ovum implantation and uneventful, successful pregnancy.

(Interestingly, Winston[22] has observed a decline in ovarian function – including a markedly reduced response to oocyte stimulation in women with a history of severe pelvic inflammatory disease).

Case II

In 1990 a middle-aged, monogamous couple, (married for 18 years) were referred to this department. Previous partner changes prior to marriage were openly discussed during joint consultation. The nulliparous female patient, aged 49, was referred (post hysterectomy) for investigation of chronic, recurrent pelvic pain which had run a variable course for most, if not all, of her marriage.

Exacerbations of female pelvic pain were specifically related to the annual surgical dilation of two "mid-penile" strictures in the male anterior urethra. This was invariably followed by a purulent urethral discharge.

All antigen detection attempts (both partners) were negative. The male MIF D-K IgG Chlamydia serology was positive at a maximum dilution 1/64.

Female serology identified an astonishing IgM response with D-K positivity to a titre of 1/1024. Extended anti-chlamydial therapy led to an eventual return of sero-negative status in both patients with a concurrent marked clinical improvement maintained throughout two years of follow-up.

These two cases illustrate several points of interest.

Concepts of chlamydial reactivation are discussed by Dr Rogstad in

Chapter 6. The unique development cycle of Chlamydia offers a plausible basis for a concept of life-long chlamydial infection in some circumstances.[13]

It is interesting to speculate (Case II):- was this pathological sequence as follows?

1. Surgical intervention in the male leading to exacerbation of long term/latent/subacute chlamydial infection (antigen-negative/sero-positive).

   Followed by:
2. Exacerbation of chronic chlamydial-induced pelvic pain in the female partner.

±
3. Delayed hypersensitivity response. (60kDa heat shock protein) ± inappropriate host immune response.

(These findings may offer some support for the hypothesis describing reactivation of latent chlamydial genital infection described by Dr R S Morton in Chapter 14.)

The application of Chlamydia serology in couples who are both experiencing features of long term/chronic chlamydial genital tract disease may be more relevant than isolated application of Chlamydia serology in individual patients, whatever the stage of disease dissemination.

Case II is particularly unusual. IgM antibody production at very high titres,with a 6-fold reduction in dilution following three months of antichlamydial therapy has not previously been seen.

IgM is rarely identified. In the serology study (discussed previously),[10] of 7,002 cases attending Genito Urinary Medicine IgM was detected in only 2.6% of the cases, of which 98% related to *C. trachomatis* D-K.

The low prevalence of IgM in this study compared with other series was thought to be due to the inclusion of a large number of cases with chronic genital infections.

The only other serological study we have undertaken which identified significant numbers of D-K IgM positive subjects referred to a series of women patients who were treated for infertility.

They were recipients of donated semen prior to the screening of donors for genital tract Chlamydia D-K.[23]

IS SEROLOGY A DIAGNOSTIC TEST?

This question merits further discussion.

The majority of GUM specialists and microbiologists consider serology tests of little value for the diagnosis of current CTGI, because of its low specificity. This claim is based on the following findings or assumptions:

Presence of chlamydia IgG in a large number of patients with no clinical, epidemiological or microbiological evidence of being infected with chlamydial antigen

In these studies, the serology tests used were either EIA or indirect immunofluorescence (IFT) using a single antigen such as LGV prototype strains. Other studies have shown that these tests mostly detect cross-reactive and group-specific Chlamydia IgG and that IgG to CTDK accounts for only half of the IgG detected. The remaining IgG detected is related to nongenital *C. pneumoniae* or *C. psittaci*. The results of these studies clearly indicate that commonly used single antigen serology tests such as EIA and IFT lack the ability to differentiate IgG to CTDK from IgG to non-genital Chlamydia species and as such produce a large number of false positive results.

Poor correlation between the presence of IgG in blood and presence of chlamydial antigen in the genital tract

In chlamydial genital infection, the specificity of serology tests is being compared with the presence/absence of chlamydial antigen in the genital tract. We believe that these two tests should not be compared with each other, because of fundamental differences in their sensitivity for detecting IgG or chlamydial antigen during the natural history of CTGI. Antigen detection tests are most sensitive in patients with acute and early infection and least sensitive in those with chronic, recurrent or asymptomatic disease. In contrast, type-specific serology tests are less sensitive during the acute stage of CTGI and most sensitive in patients with chronic disease.

The assumption that IgG generally represents past infection

Our studies of contacts refute such an assumption, because

a) in nearly half of the contacts with IgG at a level or 1/16 of higher, chlamydial antigen was also detected in their genital tract, indicating that at least in about half of the IgG positive contacts, the presence of IgG is a true indicator of a current CTGI.

b) In approximately two thirds of contacts with IgG levels of 1/64 to 1/256, chlamydial antigen was also present in their genital tract. This finding confirms results of previous studies that the presence of IgG at a level of 1/64 or higher is a reliable indicator of current CTGI.

Studies have shown that CTGI is naturally a chronic disease with a very low rate of spontaneous recovery and that without treatment infection may persist for several years
These findings may suggest that in patients with symptoms of non specific genital infections (NSGI) who have not been treated, the presence of IgG may indicate a current CTGI.

Based on our studies and experience it is suggested that a cost effective and efficient strategy for maximising diagnosis, efficacy of treatment and population control of CTGIs could be achieved by a combination of both antigen detection tests and type specific serology.

Test selection criteria would include duration of exposure/infection, presence or absence of symptoms, and previous treatment/absence of treatment. The contact tracing of D-K IgG positive, antigen negative individuals may well be justified.

CONCLUSION

The protected intra-cellular environment in which Chlamydiae are metabolically active, together with the presence of a metabolically inactive component of the developmental cycle may afford protection against host defence mechanisms, as well as against anti-chlamydial therapy. This means that absolute and complete eradication of chlamydial disease with antimicrobial therapy may be more difficult to achieve than is widely conceptualised. It may also provide an explanation for subsequent development of both asymptomatic and recurrent chronic infection.

There is potential for the continued presence of inert organisms to provide an opportunity for future recrudescence. This occurs in all chlamydial diseases. In the case of serovars D-K it is not always easy to differentiate whether a recurrence has been endogenously or exogenously acquired.

We cannot escape the widespread belief that Chlamydia serology is regarded by many eminent authorities on the subject to be of limited diagnostic significance. The application of test systems based on individual serovars could be a way forward.

Whilst recognising that Human papillomavirus (HPV) infection has been established as a cause of cervical cancer, epidemiological studies suggest that *C. trachomatis* infection also confers increased risk for cervical squamous cell carcinoma (SCC). Whether this risk is serotype specific is unknown.

An example of individual serovar investigation has recently been published by Anttila *et al*[24]. This is believed to be the first study providing longitudinal seroepidemiological evidence of an association between specific serotypes of *C. trachomatis* and cervical SCC. It was demonstrated that the presence of serum IgG antibodies to *C. trachomatis* serotype G was associated with the highest risk of developing SCC. It is suggested that exposure to *C. trachomatis* takes place several years or even decades before the diagnosis of cervical SCC.

The link between bacterial infections and carcinogenesis is not clear.

Release of nitric oxide and the specific inhibition of host cell apoptosis by *C. trachomatis* may be possible mechanisms occurring in chronic chlamydial infections that could initiate or promote cervical carcinogenesis.

It was stated that future studies should address the question of whether there are any specific determinants related to serotype G that may be directly or indirectly carcinogenic.

The work cited in this chapter suggests that species specific Chlamydia serology is a useful adjunct to antigen detection.

Future serological studies and developments may well complement modern diagnostic endeavours. Improved speed and efficiency of contact tracing the infected female or male partner may decrease recurrence rates, especially of male urethral infection and reduce the burden of disseminated disease. The potential for improvement in diagnosis before treatment is attractive to clinicians as well as to patients.

It is valid to argue for the wider application of MIF Chlamydia serology in both individuals and couples. There should be particular emphasis on serial monitoring over time in those patients with early recurrences, suspected latency or with clinical evidence of disseminated, subacute or chronic disease.

This chapter opened by asking the question:- "Is there a role for serology in genital chlamydial disease?" The answer has to be in the affirmative, especially if further clinical research and technological developments are pursued.

REFERENCES

1. Oriel JD. (1986) The Carrier State. *Chlamydia trachomatis. J Antimicrobiol Chemother* **18** (Supplement A): 67–71.

2. Schachter J. (1999) Infection and Disease Epidemiology in Chlamydia – Intracellular Biology, Pathogenesis and Immunity. Ed Stephens RS. ASM Press. Chapter 6, 154–157.

3. Howell MR, Quinn TC, Braithwaite W. *et al.* (1998). Screening women for *Chlamydia trachomatis* in family planning clinics – the cost-effectiveness of DNA amplification assays. *Sex Trans Dis* 108–117.

4. Clay JC, Bowman CA. (1996). Controlling chlamydial Infection. *Genito Urinary Medicine* **72:** 145.

5. Pimenta J, Catchpole M, Gray M *et al* (2000). Screening for Genital Chlamydial Infection. *Br Med J* **321:** 629–631.

6. Treharne JD, Darougar S, Jones BR. (1977). Modification of the micro-immunofluorescence test to provide a routine serodiagnostic test for chlamydial infection. *J Clin Pathol* **30:** 510–517.

7. Thomas K, Coughlin L, Mannion PT, Haddad NG. (2000). The value of *Chlamydia trachomatis* antibody testing as part of routine fertility investigation. *Human Reproduction* **15**(5): 1079–1082.

8. Moss TR, Hawkswell J. (1987). Clinical and Microbiological Investigation of Women with Acute Salpingitis and their Consorts. *Br J Obstet Gynaecol* **94:** 187–188.

9. Moss TR, Hawkswell J. (1986). Evidence of Infection with *Chlamydia trachomatis* in Patients with Pelvic Inflammatory Disease: Value of Partner Investigation. *Fertility and Sterility.* March 429–430.

10. Moss TR, Darougar S, Woodland R *et al.* (1993). Antibodies to Chlamydia Species in Patients Attending a Genitourinary Clinic and the Impact of Antibodies to C. *pneumoniae* and C. *psittaci* on the Sensitivity and the Specificity of *C. trachomatis* serology tests. *Sex Trans Dis* **20**(2): 61–65.

11. Moss TR, Darougar S. Sensitivity, specificity and predictive values of symptoms, culture and serological tests for indicating a current chlamydial genital infection in contacts. Unpublished data.

12. Ward ME. (1999). Mechanisms of Chlamydia-induced disease. The Role of chlamydial Heat Shock Proteins in the Pathogenesis of Disease in Chlamydia – Intracellular Biology, Pathogenesis and Immunity. Ed Stephens RS. ASM Press. Chapter 7. 186–187.

13. Morton RS, Kinghorn GK. (1999). Genitourinary chlamydial infection: a reappraisal and hypothesis. *Int J of STD & AIDS* **10:** 765–775.

14. Taylor-Robinson D. (1991). Genital Chlamydial Infections: Clinical aspects, diagnosis, treatment and prevention in: Recent Advances in Sexually Transmitted diseases and AIDS 4. Editors: Harris JRW, Forster SM, Churchill Livingstone.

15. Rank RG. (1999). Models of Immunity in Chlamydia – Intracellular Biology, Pathogenesis and Immunity. Ed. Stephens RS. ASM Press Chapter 9. 239–295.

16. Brunham RC. (1999) Human Immunity to Chlamydiae in Chlamydia – Intracellular Biology, Pathogenesis and Immunity. Ed Stephen RS. ASM Press. Chapter 8. 211–238.

17. Personal communication.

18. Rowland GF, Forsey T, Moss TR. *et al.* (1985). Failure of *in vitro* Fertilization and Embryo Replacement following infection with *Chlamydia trachomatis. J in vitro Fert and Embryo Transfer.* **2**(3): 151–155.

19. Rowland GF, Moss TR. (1985). *In Vitro* Fertilization. Previous Ectopic Pregnancy and *Chlamydia trachomatis* infection. Letter to the Editor. *Lancet.* **11:** 8459

20. Moss TR, Rowland GF. Fothergill D *et al.* (1985). Is the incidence of ectopic pregnancy rising? Letter to Editor *Br Med J* 26.10.85.

21. Moss TR, Steptoe PC. (1984). *Chlamydia trachomatis*: Importance of *in-vitro* fertilization? *J Royal Soc Med* **77:** 70–72.

22. Personal communication

23. Moss TR, Nicholls A, Viercant P. *et al.* (1986). *Chlamydia trachomatis* and Infertility. Letter to the Editor *Lancet* **II:** 8501 p218.

24. Anttila T, Saikku P *et al.* (2001). Serotypes of *Chlamydia trachomatis* and Risk for Development of Cervical Squamous Cell Carcinoma. *JAMA* **285:** 47–51.

CHAPTER 5

Therapeutic management

Janette Clarke
Pinderfields and Pontefract Hospitals NHS Trust, Wakefield, UK

INTRODUCTION

In this chapter, studies of therapy for uncomplicated and complicated genital infections with *Chlamydia trachomatis* serovars D-K will be appraised with reference to our knowledge of the lifecycle of the organism and theoretical knowledge of antibiotic sites of action. Factors in assessing microbiological and clinical cure will be discussed. Consideration will be given to treatment options in pregnancy and the potential induction of latent disease by certain antibiotics. Current recommended regimes will be compared, and prospects for improving therapeutic management will be discussed.

THE AIM OF THERAPY IN GENITAL CHLAMYDIAL INFECTIONS

The twin goals of microbiological clearance and clinical cure are obvious aims in any symptomatic patient. However, many people infected with Chlamydia have no symptoms, and their partners may or may not be infected. It is this practice of treating asymptomatic cases or contacts of infection that reinforces the need for safe and effective therapy with minimal side effects.

THE LIFE CYCLE OF CHLAMYDIA AND ANTIBIOTICS

An understanding of the unique reproductive cycle of Chlamydiae gives the theoretical basis for therapy. The elementary bodies (EBs) transform to reticulate bodies (RBs); RBs divide and finally differentiate back to EBs, which are released by host cell lysis. The metabolic activity within cells means that antibiotics must achieve sufficient intracellular tissue levels to be effective. The whole cycle takes about 40 hours in culture systems; this slow life cycle implies that a long course (over 5 days) of therapy is required or high tissue levels from a single dose therapy must be maintained over such a period. Tetracyclines, azithromycin, ofloxacin and erythromycin work to interfere with chlamydial protein synthesis.

PENICILLINS AND CHLAMYDIA

Penicillin and other beta-lactam antibiotics inhibit the growth of peptidoglycan-containing bacteria by specific inhibition of penicillin binding proteins. Mycoplasmas lack peptidoglycan and are refractory to penicillin. Chlamydiae share some structural features with mycoplasmas; however, Chlamydiae are interrupted in their life cycle by penicillin. Recent genomic analysis[1] indicates that Chlamydiae have the capacity to synthesise peptidoglycan. There is considerable controversy in microbiological circles about whether the walls of chlamydial elementary bodies contain peptidoglycans. The ultrastructural changes associated with penicillin use include the development of abnormal enlarged reticulate bodies. These abnormal forms have a low expression of outer membrane proteins, which may diminish immune recognition and clearance, but maintain intracellular survival - a recipe for latent infection[2].

IN VITRO STUDIES

In laboratory tests that evaluate the growth of Chlamydiae in cell cultures[3,4,5] the tetracyclines, erythromycin, rifampicin, certain fluoroquinolones (especially ofloxacin) and azithromycin are all highly active against these organisms. Sulphonamides and clindamycin are also active against *C. trachomatis*, but to a lesser degree. Penicillin and ampicillin suppress chlamydial multiplication but do not eradicate the organism *in vitro*. The cephalosporins appear to be relatively ineffective and streptomycin, gentamicin, neomycin, kanamycin, vancomycin, ristocetin, spectinomycin, and nystatin are not effective at concentrations inhibitory for most bacteria and fungi.

There does not appear to be much strain-to-strain variation in susceptibility to antibiotics. Antimicrobial resistance in Chlamydiae has been described in one small clinical study in the past year in the USA[6], but has not been reported from any other centre. Thus antimicrobial susceptibility testing is not recommended in the current routine management of patients with chlamydial infection.

ESTABLISHED DRUGS IN PRACTICE

Characteristics of ideal anti-chlamydial therapies are listed in **Box 1**
   Current options for therapy will be discussed by antibiotic class.

Tetracyclines
These are bacteriostatic agents, which interfere with bacterial protein synthesis.
   There is equivalent therapeutic action of tetracycline, doxycycline and minocycline, but doxycycline is preferred because of less frequent dosing, fair side effect profile and fewer dietary restrictions. Tetracycline, minocycline and doxycycline have all been shown to eradicate *C. trachomatis* from male urethra (as judged by culture) with failure rates of between 0-3% with 7, 14 or 21 days therapy[3]; in women cervical infections had declared failure rates of 0-8% in similar studies. Single doses are not effective. However, Reedy[7] demonstrated that a 3-day course of doxycycline at standard dosage (100mg twice daily) was equivalent in outcome to a 7-day course in women with uncomplicated chlamydial cervicitis, as judged by three-week post therapy PCR screening.

Box 1. Ideal Characteristics of treatments for genital Chlamydia

- Microbiological cure - at least 95% efficacy
- Effective in both clinically apparent and asymptomatic infection
- Safe in clinical practice
- Ease of dosing - single dose preferable
- Minimal disturbance of patient lifestyle
- Minimal side effects
- Safe in pregnancy
- Cost effective, low cost
- Occasional missed dosages in a multi-dose regimen not significant
- Agent(s) treat concomitant infections e.g. gonorrhoea

Side effects of doxycycline are commonly gastrointestinal, with up to 20% compliant patients complaining of nausea and vomiting. Calcium, iron and magnesium containing medications should not be taken with tetracyclines because they interfere with absorption. Food interferes with the absorption of all tetracyclines except minocycline and doxycycline.

Twice daily doxycycline has been shown to have better compliance than tetracycline taken four times daily. Minocycline is less favoured since it is associated with vestibular toxicity, and is more expensive than doxycycline. Triple tetracycline (Deteclo) is probably as good as doxycycline; photosensitisation is more common with Deteclo, and there is little data on efficacy if compliance is poor.

Oxytetracycline at a dose of 250mg four times daily for 7 days has been shown to be effective in limited evidence, but the effects of missing doses is not documented.

Tetracyclines are contraindicated in established or suspected pregnancy and in children under 8 years old because of discolouration of permanent teeth and disturbance of growth in developing bone.

Doxycycline 100mg twice daily for 7 days is a standard therapy with which all new antibiotic regimens have been compared[4,5]

Macrolides
Erythromycin, clarithromycin and azithromycin from this group will be considered. They are bacteriostatic agents that inhibit bacterial protein synthesis.

Erythromycin has similar *in vitro* activity to tetracycline, but is poorly tolerated in doses shown to be clinically effective. Reported failure rates at 7 days of 0-37% in males with NGU and in non-pregnant women with cervicitis of 0-34% are poorer than with azithromycin or doxycycline. Discontinuation due to gastrointestinal upset is common. A 2g daily dose may produce adverse effects in 70% of patients. A seven-day 1g daily dose still had a 34% adverse event profile and a four-fold failure rate compared with successful 2g dosing. Longer dosing schedules such as 500mg twice daily for 14 days have reported efficacy rates between 73% and 95%. Two weeks seems more effective than 7 days at 500mg twice daily, but compliance with longer regimes is likely to be poor. Erythromycin and clarithromycin have important interactions with some drugs. They may potentiate terfenadine, for example, with the risk of ventricular arrythmias.

Clarithromycin has a longer half-life than erythromycin and has been found to be clinically safe and effective in NGU and cervicitis[8] at a dose of 250mg twice daily.

Roxithromycin 300mg daily for 7 days has equivalent effect to erythromycin.

Azithromycin has rapid and extensive penetration into intracellular tissues, with sustained levels with an estimated tissue half-life of a 500mg dose of about 60 hours. This may exceed the minimum inhibitory concentration for *C. trachomatis* by 3- to 10-fold for up to 5 days; clinical trials have been based on double this dose. Side effects are rare, with gastrointestinal upset in less than 10% subjects in reported series. Interactions are also less marked than with other macrolides.

Azithromycin is well established as single dose therapy for uncomplicated male and female infections, for NGU[9] and for treating contacts of infection. There is limited safety data on use in pregnancy. Azithromycin may be more effective for patients with erratic health seeking behaviour, and both cost and use-effectiveness studies[10,11] have demonstrated that single dose azithromycin is superior to 7 day dosing with doxycycline. Carlin and Barton[12] found that men with NGU preferred single-dose azithromycin to a seven day course of doxycycline; this approach was also found to be cost-effective since fewer treatment failures and clinic visits were recorded in those receiving azithromycin. Hillis *et al*[11] found comparable high rates of use and effectiveness between single dose azithromycin and seven days of doxycycline in a randomised controlled study of 196 women and their partners with a PCR follow-up test at four weeks. Failures in both groups were all in women with risk behaviours consistent with re-infection.

Quinolones
The fluoroquinolones, synthetic derivatives of nalidixic acid are bactericidal, inhibiting bacterial DNA gyrase. They vary in anti-chlamydial activity. Norfloxacin and ciprofloxacin are not sufficiently effective for use in suspected chlamydial infections.[13] Ofloxacin, levofloxacin, grepafloxacin, trovafloxacin and sparfloxacin have been assessed in clinical trials. Ofloxacin has been used in varying protocols. Seven-day regimens of 200mg twice daily or 400mg once daily are highly effective, but a 5-day course had a cure rate of only 20%. There are no data on whether a missed dose on the single daily routine has any effect on cure rate. However, ofloxacin is active against

mycoplasma and gonoccocal infections, making a relatively expensive group of drugs more cost effective in treating patients with simultaneous infections.

Adverse reactions are rare. Neurological disturbances, usually limited to dizziness and mood alteration, have been reported in less than 5% patients using ofloxacin. There is a concern that tendinitis may be provoked by fluoroquinolones, and this may limit their use in growing adolescents. Interactions with non-steroidal anti-inflammatory drugs may potentiate neurological side effects.

Penicillins
The debate about how and why penicillins have an effect on Chlamydiae *in vitro* has been discussed. Clinical response to penicillins is unpredictable, and penicillins have no action against ureaplasmas. Ampicillin, amoxicillin, co-amoxiclav and pivampicillin have been shown to be active clinically. Since suppression rather than elimination of infection is possible, follow-up testing is desirable but rarely documented in trials.

Amoxicillin
Amoxicillin is preferred over ampicillin for oral administration because of better absorption and fewer side effects. Meta-analysis of the use of amoxicillin in chlamydial infections in pregnancy[14] compared with erythromycin indicated a similar cure rate for the two regimens, but a much better side effect profile for amoxicillin.

OTHER ACTIVE DRUGS NOT USED IN CLINICAL PRACTICE

Rifampicin is effective against Chlamydiae, as is rifabutin. Resistance to rifampicin develops rapidly *in vitro*; and may appear during therapy.[4] This has led to a disinclination to use these drugs in clinical practice. Spiramycin has some effect *in vitro* but is not a drug of choice.

INEFFECTIVE DRUGS (Box 2)

Several classes of antibiotics in common use for urogenital infections are not effective in treating chlamydial infections. These failures may be due to the inability to reach therapeutic intracellular levels. In particular, cephalosporin based combinations for treating suspected pelvic infections should be avoided.

In a detailed study of women treated with ß-lactam antibiotics for acute salpingitis, Sweet *et al*[15] found persistence of endometrial and cervical infection despite completion of antibiotic regimes and clinical improvement.

ANTIBIOTICS ARE ONLY HALF THE STORY...

Microbiological and pharmaceutical studies may not reflect clinical practice in treating real patients. In sexual infections, the social and sexual behaviour of infected persons to be treated can have significant influence on the success of a drug regimen. Patients and partners should understand the infection and proposed therapy, the need for contact tracing, sexual abstinence and the benefits of completing treatment. The treatment should be effective, easy to take, with minimal side effects and cheap for patient and doctor.

Antibiotics chosen should have activity against other likely contemporaneous infection with gonococci, mycoplasma and ureaplasma.

Women may have particular needs from antibiotics in terms of efficacy and safety. Regimens for apparently uncomplicated infection should still show efficacy for pelvic disease. Pregnancy leads to concerns to treat effectively to abolish any risk of fetal infection at delivery.

Serious infections requiring inpatient care may mimic acute abdominal catastrophe and provoke gastrointestinal upset. Parenteral therapies should be available to those unable to tolerate oral therapy.

Patient preference and cost-effectiveness studies are becoming more important in influencing therapeutic choices in treating uncomplicated chlamydial infections.

Critical appraisal of the design of published clinical studies in treating

---

Box 2. Drugs known to be ineffective against genital chlamydial infections

- Aminoglycosides
- Sulphonamides
- Trimethoprim
- Clindamycin
- Cephalosporins

sexually transmitted infections (**Box 3**) reveals that very few fulfil such criteria. Treatment recommendations in national and international guidelines[16,17,18] are heavily based on historical and anecdotal experience, *in vitro* susceptibility testing and small trials. Most data are found on treating men with NGU. There are few studies in women with uncomplicated disease, and very small studies in pregnant women. Follow up to confirm clearance of infection have either been poorly described or limited to less than two weeks.

ASSESSING SUCCESS OF TREATMENT

The problem of assessing cure in uncomplicated Chlamydia, which is usually asymptomatic especially in women, has been compounded by the poor sensitivity of tests such as antigen detection or culture which have been used as markers of infection and tests of cure in most therapeutic trials. There are persistent therapy failure rates, whatever the drug, of 0-37%; even azithromycin has failure rates as high as 15% in some series. There may be poor absorption or bioavailability of the drugs or there may be relative or absolute resistance to treatment. Apparent failure of therapy may be due to re-infection

---

Box 3. Ideal characteristics of studies in Chlamydia therapy

- Randomised, double-blind studies of either active drug vs. placebo or between two treatments.

- Study groups reflect demographic distribution of infection in general population.

- Clear description of inclusion criteria and infection severity (symptomatic/ asymptomatic/complicated).

- Method of confirming infection declared.

- Drug dosage, duration and compliance assessments described. Sexual partners of subjects traced and treated.

- Sexual abstinence/condom use/simultaneous therapy of partners documented.

- Follow-up testing of cure clearly described in method and interval.

- Adverse reactions, discontinuations listed.

- Detailed review of persistent positive subjects to determine sexual behaviour risks for re-infection.

by sexual contact with an untreated partner rather than persistence of original infection. Many methods of ascertaining cure will be positive in the presence of non-viable organisms, and may become negative with interval re-testing.

Complicated presentation, as with pelvic infection, may be polymicrobial and clinical end points may measure efficacy against several organisms.

PROVING EFFICACY OF TREATMENT

Optimal assessment techniques should detect actively reproducing organisms at high sensitivity and specificity. Nucleic acid amplification tests have been used in studies in the past decade, but PCR and LCR cannot discriminate living from dead Chlamydiae. Transcription-mediated amplification (TMA) would now be considered the optimal test of cure, but is not clinically available in most centres.

Test of cure is recommended after completing therapy in pregnant women and those using erythromycin. Tests should be performed no earlier than 3 weeks after end of therapy. This imposes a five-week episode of sexual abstinence on the treated person. Re-testing is not needed for those treated with azithromycin or doxycycline unless re-infection is suspected or symptoms persist.

Some clinical studies have started to address the question of persistence[19]. Tests over five months from three genital sites using two sensitive polymerase chain reaction (PCR) assays for detection after seven days doxycycline in a well motivated study group were positive in only 1 of 20 study subjects; she had been re-infected.

TREATING IN PREGNANCY

In a meta-analysis of 11 small studies[14], amoxicillin and erythromycin have been found to be equally effective. End points in pregnancy are, however, different – the obvious measure is the documented prevention of neonatal infection. Unfortunately, very few studies have followed the woman to delivery and examined or treated the neonate. Guidance to perform a test of cure by culture three weeks after completion of therapy may be impractical if infection is late in term.

Neonatal treatment of clinical problems are best documented for neonatal ophthalmia. Oral erythromycin, 50mg/kg is the preferred agent, with tetracycline eye ointments having high relapse rates.

COMPLICATIONS

Pelvic inflammatory disease

As discussed in another chapter, the clinical presentation of PID lacks sensitivity and specificity. However, there is some evidence to suggest that delay in therapy is associated with increased risk of subsequent tubal infertility. A low clinical threshold to treat in any woman with undiagnosed acute or chronic pelvic pain is recommended. It is important that all empirical therapy of PID should cover three probable infections – Chlamydia, gonorrhoea and anaerobic infections. Gonococcal PID may exist in the absence of endocervical infection. Most studies of treating PID are based on inpatient gynaecological care. There are little data to suggest that milder cases managed in office or outpatient settings warrant any modification of these protocols. Intravenous access may be needed if vomiting is marked. There are recommendations that more serious cases should all receive IV antibiotics to ensure maximal efficacy but there are little supporting data. Parenteral therapy should be continued for a further 24 hours *after* sustained clinical improvement is established, before oral treatment is substituted (**Box 4**). Studies of microbial persistence in PID[15] indicate that clinical resolution may not be a reliable marker of micobiological cure. Follow-up tests should be linked to sexual abstinence until the sexual partner is treated.

Peri-hepatitis (Fitz-Hugh-Curtis syndrome) is a complication of chlamydial PID. Apart from anecdotal evidence that adhesions could be divided at diagnostic laparoscopy there is no evidence to modify therapy from PID.

Epididymo-orchitis

Empirical therapy is once again the rule, depending to some extent on the age and sexual behaviour of the man. Antibiotics should cover common urogenital pathogens, gonorrhoea and Chlamydia.

Typical recommendations include ofloxacin 200mg twice daily for 14 days, or doxycycline 100mg twice daily for 10-14 days with initial dosing of ceftriaxone 250mg IM stat, or ciprofloxacin 500mg oral stat. Test of cure is generally regarded as clinical resolution.

Prostatitis is a controversial area of therapy, since the actual etiological causation by Chlamydiae is disputed. Nevertheless, long courses of fluoroquinolones such as ofloxacin and ciprofloxacin have been shown to improve symptoms.

Box 4. Treating chlamydial PID - some suggestions

Note: Antibiotic choice against gonorrhoea should reflect local strain sensitivities. Regimes should be continued for at least 14 days, with change to oral therapy 24 hours **after** clinical improvement.

- Cefoxitin 2g tds IV plus doxycycline 100mg bd IV; continue with oral metronidazole 400mg bd plus doxycycline 100mg bd to complete 14 days' therapy

or

- Clindamycin 900mg tds IV plus gentamicin 2mg/kg IV loading dose, then 1.5 mg/kg tds; continue as above with metronidazole/doxycycline orally.

- Ofloxacin 400mg bd IV plus metronidazole 500mg tds IV.

- Cefoxitin 2g tds IV *plus* erythromycin 50mg/kg IV (in pregnancy)

Sexually Acquired Reactive Arthritis (SARA)

There is some evidence that eradicating acute chlamydial genital tract infection tends to reduce the risk of relapse in SARA. There is only one study indicating that long term therapy with anti-chlamydial antibiotics has any effect on clinical outcome[16.]

TREATING GENITAL CHLAMYDIAL INFECTION – CONCLUSIONS

There are relatively few antibiotics active against Chlamydiae (**Table 1**), and some are suspected to induce a latent infection rather than produce microbiological clearance. The complex and prolonged life cycle of these intracellular organisms requires sustained therapeutic levels of antibiotics in the target tissues. Clinical success also depends on patient adherence with effective antibiotic regimes, sexual abstinence during therapy and treating sexual partners.

Future trials of therapy should be compared with current "gold standards" of doxycycline and azithromycin. All such trials should have use- and cost-effectiveness analyses, and assess patient preferences for treatment. Tests of cure using TMA would settle the question of persistence after therapy. New agents for use in pregnancy are required to dispel disquiet around current therapies.

Table 1. Comparing effective therapies

Assessment of recommended drugs for uncomplicated genital infection with *Chlamydia trachomatis* serovars D-K (after Fitzgerald *et al*)

Drug	Advantages	Disadvantages
Doxycycline 100mg twice daily x 7 days	Efficacy > 95% Relatively cheap Missed doses do not seem to effect efficacy	Contraindicated in pregnancy Photosensitisation Side effects in 20% (gastrointestinal upset)
Deteclo 300mg twice daily x 7 days	Cheap Efficacy >95%	Cannot take with milk Contraindicated in pregnancy Photosensitivity
Azithromycin 1g stat	Efficacy >95% Once only dosing Patient preferred	Expense Limited long term follow-up data Limited data on use in pregnancy
Erythromycin 500mg four times daily x 7 days or 500mg twice daily x 14 days	Cheap Safe in pregnancy	Four times daily or lengthy dosing schedule limits compliance Efficacy<95% Significant side-effects in 25% to discontinuation
Ofloxacin 400mg daily x 7 days	Efficacy >95% Good side-effect profile	Expensive Lack of data about efficacy in missing doses Contraindicated in pregnancy Avoid in young people (risk of joint damage)
Amoxicillin 500mg three times daily x 7 days	Good side-effect profile Safe in pregnancy	Poor efficacy Risk of latency Three times daily dosing

REFERENCES

1. Chopra I, Storey C, Falla TJ, Pearce JH. (1998). Antibiotics, peptidoglycan synthesis and genomics: the chlamydial anomaly revisited. (review article 40 refs) *Microbiology* **133:** 2673–2678.
2. Morton RS, Kinghorn GR. (1999). Genitourinary chlamydial infection: a reappraisal and hypothesis. *Int J STD & AIDS* **10:** 765–775.
3. Toomey KE, Barnes RC. (1990). Treatment of *Chlamydia trachomatis* Genital Infection. *Rev Infect Dis* **12**(suppl 6): S645–655 (review article 114 refs.)
4. Weber JT, Johnson RE. (1995). New treatments for *Chlamydia trachomatis* genital infection. *Clin Infect Dis* **20**(suppl 1): S66–71.
5. Jones RB. (1991). New treatments for *Chlamydia trachomatis*. *Am J Obstet Gynaecol* **164**(6):1789–93.
6. Bhullar VB, Workowski KA, Farshy CE, Black CM. (2000). Multiple drug-resistant *Chlamydia trachomatis* associated with clinical treatment failure. *J Infect Dis* **181**(4): 1421–7.
7. Reedy MB, Sulak PJ, Miller SL, Ortiz M, Kasberg-Preece C, Kuehl TJ. (1997). Evaluation of a 3-day course of doxycycline for the treatment of uncomplicated *Chlamydia trachomatis* cervicitis. *Infect Dis Obstet Gynaecol* **5**(1): 18–22.
8. Stein GE, Mummaw NL, Havlichek DH. (1995). A preliminary study of clarithromycin versus doxycycline in the treatment of non-gonococcal urethritis and mucopurulent cervicitis. *Pharmacotherapy* **15**(6): 727–31
9. Stamm WE, Hicks CB, Martin DH *et al*. (1995). Azithromycin for empirical treatment of the non-gonococcal syndrome in men. A randomised double-blind study. *JAMA* **274:** 545–9.
10. Magdid D, Douglas JMJ, Schwartz JS. (1996). Doxycycline compared with azithromycin for treating women with genital *Chlamydia trachomatis* infection: an incremental cost-effectiveness analysis. *Ann Intern Med* **124:** 389–99.
11. Hillis SD, Coles FB, Litchfield B, Black CM, Mojica B, Schmitt K, St.Louis ME. (1998). Doxycycline and azithromycin for the prevention of chlamydial persistence or recurrence one month after treatment in women. A use-effectiveness study in public health settings. *Sex Trans Dis* **25:** 5–11.
12. Carlin EM, Barton SE. (1996). Azithromycin as the first-line treatment of nongonococcal urethritis (NGU); a study of follow-up rates, contact attendance and patients' treatment preference. *Int J STD & AIDS* **7**(3): 185–9.
13. Ziegler C, Stary A, Mailer H, Kopp W, Gebhart W, Soltz-Szots J. (1992). Quinolones as an alternative treatment of chlamydial, mycoplasmas and gonococcal urogenital infections. *Dermatology* **185**(2): 128–31.
14. Brocklehurst P, Rooney G. (2000). Interventions for treating genital *Chlamydia trachomatis* infection in pregnancy (Cochrane Review). In: *The Cochrane Library Issue 2*. Oxford: Update Software.
15. Sweet RL, Schachter J, Robbie MO. (1983). Failure of ß-lactam antibiotics to eradicate *Chlamydia trachomatis* in the endometrium despite apparent clinical cure of acute salpingitis. *JAMA* **250:** 2641–5.
16. Centers for Disease Control and Prevention.(1998). Guidelines for treatment of sexually transmitted diseases. *MMWR* **47**(No. RR-1): 49-59; also available at www.cdc.gov/mmwr
17. UK Clinical Effectiveness Guidelines. Clinical Effectiveness Group. (1999). *Sex Trans Infects.* **75**(suppl 1); also available at www.agum.org.uk
18. FitzGerald MR, Welch J, Robinson AJ, Ahmed-Jusuf IH. (1998). Clinical guidelines and standards for the management of uncomplicated genital chlamydial infection. *Int J STD & AIDS* **9:** 253–262.
19. Workowski KA, Lampe MF, Wong KG, Watts MB, Stamm WE. (1993). Long-term eradication of *Chlamydia trachomatis* genital infection after antimicrobial therapy; evidence against persistent infection. *JAMA* **270:** 2071–5.

CHAPTER 6

Partner notification and counselling

Karen E Rogstad
Department of Genitourinary Medicine,
Royal Hallamshire Hospital, Sheffield, UK

INTRODUCTION

Partner notification or contact tracing has been an integral part of the management of bacterial sexually transmitted diseases for more than 60 years both in the United Kingdom and the USA. It aims to identify often-asymptomatic cases to reduce morbidity in the individual, and reduce onward transmission. Originally used in the 19th century in the form of incarceration of prostitutes suspected of having syphilis, it was not until 1942 in the UK and 1936 in the USA that contact tracing was developed as a means of offering treatment to infected partners in order to control the spread of syphilis and gonorrhoea.

The prevalence of an STD in the community is dependent on biological features of the organism and behavioural factors of the individual[1]. The former includes efficiency of transmission and duration of infectiousness, and varies greatly between the different organisms causing sexually transmitted diseases. Behavioural factors include the rate of partner change, sexual mixing and barrier contraceptive use. As partner notification identifies asymptomatic cases, thus reducing duration of infectiousness, and may effect behavioural changes, to reduce ongoing transmission, then it would be expected that it will help in the control of STDs. Contact tracing should therefore be of benefit to the individual, their partners and to society via improving the public health.

WHAT IS PARTNER NOTIFICATION?

As defined by the World Health Organization[2], partner notification is

That public health activity in which sexual partners of individuals with HIV infection and those sharing injecting equipment are notified, counselled about their exposure and offered services.

This definition is equally applicable for other STDs.

The pressure upon an infected individual to participate in contact tracing varies from country to country, depending on the legal framework and attitudes towards the rights of individuals versus the rights of infected contacts and the public health. Even in countries with similar cultural backgrounds there can be diametrically opposing views, such as in Scandinavia. Norway and Denmark[3] provide absolute confidentiality for those infected with STDs and official contact tracing is opposed, whereas in Sweden index patients are legally obliged to name partners and contacts have a legal requirement to be tested[4]. In the United Kingdom patients are encouraged to co-operate with contact tracing but their participation is voluntary.

HOW IS IT PERFORMED?

Strategies for partner notification (PN) vary. In the UK, where the majority of STDs are managed in free, open access confidential clinics, PN is undertaken by dedicated healthcare professionals known as Health Advisors. These are usually trained nurses, social workers or occasionally individuals from other backgrounds who have received additional training.

When a man or woman is diagnosed as being infected with *Chlamydia trachomatis* details of sexual contacts should be requested, both current and previous. The length of look-back time varies according to the STD, but for Chlamydia would usually be all partners in the previous 3-6 months, or 4-6 weeks for symptomatic men. If there have been no partners in this time then the last partner in 6 months should be determined, although some studies suggest that this should be up to one year or longer.

Partner notification consists of three types:

Patient referral The index case is given one or more contact slips to pass on to sexual partners. This has on it the date, diagnosis, clinic, and index case's clinic number. In order to maintain confidentiality the diagnosis is indicated by a national code (which is part of a coding system, that is standardised throughout the United Kingdom and Ireland).

Provider referral The healthcare worker contacts the sexual partner. This may be done by telephone, letter or home visit, and this system is utilised when the index case will not see the contact again, wishes anonymity or is worried about the threat of violence.

Conditional referral Initial PN is undertaken by the patient with the agreement that if the contact has not attended within a specific time then provider notification will be undertaken.

Partner notification is discussed as soon as the individual is given a positive diagnosis of Chlamydia. It may be undertaken by doctor, nurse or more usually by the health advisor.

It is important that it is undertaken in a non-judgmental fashion and that confidentiality is guaranteed. The patient or index case should be reassured that neither his or her identity nor diagnosis would be disclosed during provider referral. They should be encouraged to disclose both regular and non-regular partners. As much information that is available on the contact should be elicited including name, address, telephone number, and if full details are unavailable, then a description may be useful.

Contacts can be divided into one of three groups:

Treated Partners who have been documented as already having attended for diagnosis, received treatment and not had unprotected sexual intercourse with the untreated index case since their treatment.

Contacts to be sought Some of these will prove to be untraceable if details are incomplete or incorrect.

Untraceable Partners who cannot be notified because their name and/or whereabouts are unknown, or because they are abroad and un-contactable.

An agreement should be made as to which type of PN is to be undertaken and this may vary for each contact. It needs to be accepted that in some rare cases the risk of violence to patient or health advisor may be such that partner notification is not performed. In practice there is usually a way around this, by delaying PN in order to obscure the identity of the index, and the use of letters or phone calls without home visits. Patients ought to be seen again in order to determine that contacts have been notified and received screening and treatment. The index case may also have managed to find out or be prepared to disclose additional information on contacts during the follow-up visit.

When a patient attends with a contact slip, details of their treatment and date of attendance should be noted and the slip returned to the issuing clinic.

Partner notification needs to be tailored to cultural needs[5] and access to healthcare systems, and the UK system may not be applicable to the developing world.

DOES PARTNER NOTIFICATION WORK?

There have been few properly conducted studies to assess the efficacy of contact tracing either for *C. trachomatis* or any other sexually transmitted disease. There is certainly a benefit at the individual level as a means of preventing re-infection or diagnosing individuals with previously unrecognised infection. However at a population level, as a public health intervention, the efficaciousness of partner notification is less clear, both as a means of reducing prevalence of infection in the community and reducing incidence of complications. There is even less data on cost-effectiveness and cost-benefit. Comparing studies on partner notification is fraught with difficulties, as healthcare systems vary according to country and different criteria for success are used. There is also the added difficulty that the incidence and prevalence of the infection in the community is usually not accurately known.

The Tyneside Scheme[6] which introduced a system of education and contact tracing for gonorrhoea in the north east of England resulted in an almost fourfold increase in named contacts within six months of its introduction and 25 years after its inception gonorrhoea rates in the area were 80% of the national prevalence. However other variables may have effected this difference. The proportion of contacts notified or attending for treatment is very variable, but can be high. In Indianapolis, for example, 82% of contacts of patients with gonorrhoea, Chlamydia or related conditions were contacted[7]. However many medical practitioners do not undertake PN nor refer patients to a service that do. Some General Practice studies have shown only 13% of patients would be referred to a Genito-urinary clinic for contact tracing[8] whereas in other studies GPs refer more than 50%[9]. In practices where there is no referral to an STD service for PN, contact tracing is undertaken in only a minority[10].

There is little data on the most effective method of partner notification. A systematic review of the efficacy of differing PN strategies in the management of STDs revealed only a small number of studies which met their criteria, and of these only five were methodologically strong[11]. Their limited conclusions were that:

i.   Provider referral was more efficacious than patient notification for HIV infection
ii. There was weak evidence that provider notification was better than conditional referral for syphilis
iii. Evidence was conflicting for gonorrhoea and Chlamydia.

One strong study has shown that, for NSU, provider referral is more efficacious than patient referral. However conditional and provider notification is between 4 and 8 times more expensive than patient referral[7].

In one study on cost effectiveness, a hypothetical model suggested that in the prevention of chlamydial PID contact tracing would be cost effective only if 43% of the named male partners of female cases, or 11% of the named female partners of male index cases received treatment[12]. This study did not take into account the prevention of onward transmission therefore the true cost-effectiveness is likely to have been underestimated.

WHAT ARE THE DISADVANTAGES?

There has been little work done to evaluate the psychological and social effects of partner notification. There may violence, breakdown of relationships and anxiety or depression. These may be preventable by careful discussion and counselling.

WHAT COUNSELLING SHOULD BE GIVEN?

Patients must be made aware of the sexually transmitted nature of their infection. There should be a clear discussion of the long latent period in some people and that sexual partners can be infected but asymptomatic. The possibility of complications needs to be raised, highlighting that these can occur in those who have no symptoms. Patients must also be made aware of the risk of re-infection from untreated partners, and that it can be acquired *de novo* from new partners.

Women, particularly those with chlamydial pelvic inflammatory disease, should be informed of the risk of ectopic pregnancy and further episodes of PID (which may be CT negative) and advised on accessing healthcare quickly if complications develop. The patient should be made aware of the future risk of infertility, particularly if re-infection with Chlamydia occurs.

It is essential that the patient is given time to ask questions and reassured about any anxieties they may have. In some cases referral to a clinical psychologist may be necessary.

All patients should be advised on sexual abstinence until they and their partner have been treated and a test of cure performed if appropriate. There should be education about safer sex and a demonstration of condom use where necessary.

Partner notification remains an integral part of the control of *C. trachomatis* in developed countries In the developing world PN may not be feasible because of cost, cultural barriers and stigmatisation of those with infection. Additionally the value of contact tracing where syndromic management of STDs occurs is unclear. The relevance in the 21st century with the real possibility of population screening by highly sensitive DNA amplification methods needs to be ascertained. Until there is evidence to the contrary, it should retain its key role in the management of anyone diagnosed with *C. trachomatis*. PN should follow clearly developed protocols with regular auditing of its effectiveness and be tailored to take into account the cultural differences of patients.

Acknowledgements.
I would like to thank Gill Bell and Robbie Morton for their helpful advice on the manuscript.

REFERENCES

1. Heathcote HW, Yoke JA. (1984). Gonorrhoea: transmission dynamics and control *Biomathematics* **56:** 1–105.
2. WHO Consultation document SHO/BPA/ESR/89/2.
3. Blaxter M. (1991). AIDS: World-wide policies and problems: London Office of Health Economics.
4. Thelin I, Wennstrom AM, Mardh PA. (1980). Contact tracing in patients with genital chlamydial infection *Br J Vener Dis* **56:** 259–62.
5. Mulvey G. (1995). Contact tracing and sexually transmitted disease among Aboriginal men on the Anangu Pitjantjatjara Lands *Aust J Public Health* **19:** 596–601.
6. Wigfield AS. (1972). 27 years of uninterrupted contact tracing: The 'Tyneside Scheme' *Br J Vener Dis* **48:** 37–50.

7. Katz BP, Danes CS, Quinn TS *et al.* (1998). Efficiency and cost effectiveness of field follow-up for patients with *Chlamydia trachomatis* infection in a Sexually Transmitted Disease Clinic. *Sex Trans Dis* **15:** 11–16.

8. Ross JDC, Sutherland S, Copi J. (1996). Genital *Chlamydia trachomatis* infections in primary care *Br Med J* **313:** 1992–3.

9. Rogstad KE, Kinghorn GR, Horton M. (2000). Community control of *Chlamydia trachomatis Int J STD & AIDS* **11:** 248–249.

10. Rogstad KE , Davies A, Krishna Murthy S, Searle S, Mee RA. The management of *Chlamydia trachomatis*: combined community and hospital study (In press)

11. Oxman AD, Scott E AF, Sellors JW *et al.* (1994). Partner notification for sexually transmitted diseases: an overview of the evidence. *Can J Public Health* suppl 1: S41.

12. Howell MR, Kassler WJ, Haddix A. (1997). Partner notification to prevent pelvic inflammatory diseases in women *Sex Trans Dis* **24:** 287–92.

CHAPTER 7

Complications of Chlamydia trachomatis *infection in men*

David Hicks

Royal Hallamshire Hospital, Sheffield, UK

Chlamydia trachomatis derives its name from the Latin, meaning "to cloak". This term not only describes its life-style as an obligate intracellular energy parasite but also the way in which it hides from health professionals and patients.

Around 70% of women and 50% of men are asymptomatic when infected genitally but such estimates depend on the diagnostic methodology used. Screening for the organism is not generally employed and estimations of prevalence are always an underestimate. In 1997 the UK Health Education Authority carried out a poll which showed that only 27% of adults knew what Chlamydia was.

The organism, therefore, is aided by ignorance, mis-diagnosis and inadequacies in diagnostic methods and may truly be termed a "hidden epidemic".

This chapter describes asymptomatic, symptomatic and complicated chlamydial disease in men (management and therapy is dealt with elsewhere) but first it is important to recognise that spontaneous clearance in untreated patients is possible. Just as no organism is 100% infectious then similarly its host can resist infection through a variety of mechanisms and can cope with early and established infection.

SPONTANEOUS CLEARANCE

A study[1] from a population attending a sexually transmitted infection (STI) clinic in Birmingham, Alabama is illustrative. The study group consisted of patients who had had positive cultures for _C. trachomatis_ and who then had repeat specimens performed within 45 days of initial observation, but who did not receive recommended therapy for this infection in the interval between the 2 tests. Of 74 evaluable patients, 24 (32%) had negative follow-up cultures. These cultures were tested with direct immuno-fluorescence (DFA) and polymerase chain reaction (PCR) assays for Chlamydia and 3 of the 24 (13%) proved positive. The rates of culture positivity declined significantly with increasing age and also duration of follow-up. Whilst Benzathene Penicillin resulted in apparent resolution of infection in 9 of 10 remaining patients, treatment with a cephalosporin, Metronidazole or anti-fungal agents in others was not associated with clearance of infection. Overall, in this retrospective study, resolution of _C. trachomatis_ infection occurred in 28% of 74 patients who did not receive currently recommended therapy. These data should be borne in mind when considering public health measures to control the infection as well as for proper interpretation of prevalence rates.

ASYMPTOMATIC INFECTIONS

Generally a milder urethritis is caused by _C. trachomatis_ as compared to _Neisseria gonorrhoea_. This and asymptomatic carriage of Chlamydia can be explained by host immune defences to the organism.

The incidence of asymptomatic infections would appear to be rising. This may be due to variables such as the sensitivity and specificity of tests used over time, comparability of populations studied and the depth of questioning taken in a sexual history.

In the 1970's when culture was used for diagnosis 0 – 5% of men without obvious urethritis had Chlamydia isolated.

In studies in the 1980's using enzyme immuno-assay (EIA) male asymptomatic carriage was usually found to be around 50%.

With techniques now available such as PCR which are highly sensitive and highly specific, one can expect that asymptomatic infection in men will be found to be no less and probably more common than this. In a recent study[2] of 2,308 teenage boys tested by urine ligase chain reaction test 143 (6.2%) were shown to be infected with over 90% of these being worryingly asymptomatic.

Males who are asymptomatic or who have mild urethritis tend to ignore symptoms longer than do men with obvious problems, remaining sexually active (and infective) for a longer duration without diagnosis and treatment. The fact that these men are more likely to have a long-term persistence of this organism means they may be more at risk of developing symptomatic urethritis and/or one of its complications.

Pharyngeal infection has been little studied but may be 3-6% of the STI clinic population. An absence of symptoms is probably its usual (non-) presentation in this area. One study in the UK[3] showed a prevalence of 2.4% in STI patients (only 3 cases) which were all culture negative, asymptomatic and diagnosed by PCR.

C. trachomatis was isolated from the rectum of asymptomatic homosexuals attending an STI clinic in 6% of men who practised passive rectal intercourse[4].

URETHRITIS

Both *C. trachomatis* and *N. gonorrhoea* produce clinical signs and symptoms due to their preference to infect columnar or transitional epithelium. For both, urethritis is the commonest presentation, although the epididymis, rectum and conjunctiva can also be sites of infection in men. Urethritis may be noted only as a historical event in men who have subsequently developed complications.

The inflammation produced by *C. trachomatis* is revealed as a discharge appearing at the urethral meatus with or without meatal inflammation. Symptoms experienced by the patient include discharge, burning on micturition or an itching sensation meatally or in the urethra. Discharge tends to be less acute, profuse and purulent than in men with gonococcal urethritis and has a longer incubation period (usually 7–21 days) but differences are qualitative rather than quantitative and as such, are not helpful in diagnosis.

Frequency, urgency, nocturia, haematuria, perineal pain, scrotal swelling, inguinal lymphadenopathy, pain on opening the bowels and fever can occur but are all very unusual.

Clinical evidence of urethritis depends upon the demonstration (in two or more of five fields) of urethral leucocytosis (equal to or greater than 5 polymorphonuclear leucocytes per x 1,000 field) on a Gram-stained slide of urethral secretions. This is accepted by most authorities as the benchmark of urethral inflammation but some use 10 such cells.

A polymorphonuclear leucocytosis may also be detected in the sediment of a first voided urine. The patient should not have passed urine for 4 hours prior to the test, or preferably overnight where symptoms are few or absent. The first 10-20ml of urine voided is collected and centrifuged at 400g for 5 minutes. Sediment can be removed by a sterile plastic or platinum loop for culture and Gram staining.

Leucocytosis will not reveal the presence of *C. trachomatis*, but can demonstrate its effect as inflammation. Microscopy may also differentiate gonococcal from non-gonococcal urethritis with high degrees of specificity and sensitivity in the hands of microscopists experienced in sexually transmitted disease populations.

EPIDIDYMITIS

Many organisms are implicated as causes of acute or chronic epididymitis. In keeping with its mode of transmission, *C. trachomatis* is a major cause of acute epididymitis in populations at risk of acquiring sexually transmitted infections. Pathogens such as coliforms and pseudomonads are important causes in older men, where there is often a history of urological disease or instrumentation. The original studies suggesting this association with Chlamydia used an age cut-off of 35 years of age. A good (sexual) history is a more sensitive determinant.

Classically then, the patient is a young man who may have had a urethritis (perhaps asymptomatic) who presents with a unilateral scrotal pain, swelling and tenderness accompanied by fever. The clinical and historical features are again of little help when differentiating between gonococcal, chlamydial and other bacterial aetiologies.

If the patient is not recognised as a contact of Chlamydia, or presents as the "acute scrotum", Colour Doppler Imaging is the study of choice in evaluating the condition. Its superior resolution will help to differentiate causes such as torsion of the spermatic cord, epididymal and testicular inflammation and scrotal trauma. It requires a degree of operator experience, sensitive Doppler ultrasound equipment and the operator should have knowledge of the limitations of its use.

Additional clinical information can be identified by observations of pyuria, positive bacterial culture, leukocytosis, accelerated erythrocyte sedimentation rate and a positive C-reactive protein test.

A review of histological, immunohistochemical and clinicopathological findings in chlamydial and bacterial epididymitis[5] has been performed. chlamydial epididymitis is characterised by its minimally destructive, periductal and intraepithelial inflammation with active epithelial proliferation. *E. coli* is remarkable for its highly destructive nature, forming large abscesses and xanthogranulomas.

Whilst women with pelvic inflammatory disease are counselled with reference to their subsequent fertility, our lack of knowledge and the (usually) unilateral nature of infection leads to difficulties in extending the same courtesy to men with epididymitis. It is known however that such infection can have a negative impact on sperm quality.

PROSTATITIS

Acute prostatitis is characterised by pyrexia, feverish chills, general malaise, frequency of micturition and occasionally acute retention of urine. A non-acute syndrome exists with less fulminant symptoms. Disturbances of bladder function are common including dribbling of urine post micturition and a urethral discharge may co-exist.

Suprapubic dull aching sometimes radiating to the perineal area, inguinal region, testes and penis is not uncommon with post ejaculatory pain and haematospermia said to be more frequent in non-bacterial prostatitis.

The methods for detecting urethral and prostatic inflammation in patients with chronic prostatitis have been reviewed[6] to show that first void or mid-stream urine examination has low sensitivity for detecting urethral inflammation. Examining both expressed prostatic secretions and post prostatic massage urine proves best for detecting inflammation in prostatic fluid. Combining a urethral smear with lower urinary tract localisation in the form of a Meares-Stamey four glass urine test, represents an optimal approach for detecting urethral and prostatic inflammation.

Chronic prostatitis is associated with increased blood flow to the prostatic capsule and diffuse flow through the prostatic parenchyma. Colour Doppler Ultrasonography can provide objective documentation of such abnormalities.

There remains, however, no absolute evidence that *C. trachomatis* is a cause of prostatitis. Early studies showed only around 10% of patients with non-bacterial prostatitis to have antibodies to *C. trachomatis* in serum or expressed prostatic secretions with none having the organism recovered by culture. Some men with prostatitis respond to drugs, which are active against *C. trachomatis* and where other pathogens are not found. *C. trachomatis*, however, is not thought to infect glandular tissue such as the prostate.

One mechanism used to explain the association is that the syndrome is, in part, caused by a hyper-sensitivity reaction to the organism. Some men with chronic non-bacterial prostatitis are more likely than controls to show positive delayed hypersensitivity skin test reaction to the organism[7]. A reduction in the skin test response following Azithromycin treatment goes some way to support this hypothesis.

Whilst Chlamydia has been recovered from expressed prostatic secretions in men with acute non-gonococcal urethritis and the prostatic fluid of men with non-bacterial prostatitis the definition of prostatitis used in these studies has been disputed. *C. trachomatis* has been cultured from expressed prostatic secretions of 6 men with negative urethral cultures[8].

In a study using trans-rectal biopsy of the prostate in 30 men with known positive urethral cultures for Chlamydia and a diagnosis of prostatitis (prostatic tenderness and swelling on digital examination per rectum) Chlamydia was cultured from a third of these[9]. Urethral contamination is a concern, however.

In an attempt to overcome this, a study was performed using ultrasound-directed percutaneous biopsies but this was unable to isolate the organism from any specimen although it did find a chronic inflammatory reaction in the majority of cases[10].

Chlamydial DNA has been found in 4 out of 135 prostatic biopsies using PCR in a study excluding men with microscopically diagnosed urethritis or other evidence of infection with gonorrhoea, Chlamydia or ureaplasma[11].

PROCTITIS

Intestinal involvement is well described in *Lymphogranuloma venereum* (LGV) infection and it can cause a severe proctitis. The oculogenital serovars of Chlamydia can also produce proctitis but this tends to be of a milder nature or even asymptomatic.

The condition is characterised by ano-rectal pain, a bloody mucopurulent discharge, tenesmus and diarrhoea.

With naked eye inspection, the proctitis can take on a granular appearance, but this may be absent. Many infected individuals are diagnosed only during routine diagnostic testing for STIs.

Sigmoidoscopy may be normal or can reveal mild inflammatory changes with small erosions and/or follicles in the lower 10cm of the rectum.

Histologically, rectal biopsy shows polymorphonuclear leucocyte infiltrate within the lamina propria with giant cells, crypt abscesses and granulomas often present.

It may be difficult, on the evidence of histopathological findings, to differentiate this from Crohn's Disease or unexplained proctitis. Where inflammatory bowel disease in a homosexual patient is suspected, chlamydial infection should be considered.

A small number of faecal leucocytes may be present on microscopy but the test is not sensitive enough to indicate proctitis.

The diagnosis of chlamydial proctitis is made by isolation or detection of the organism from the rectum and a response to symptoms with appropriate therapy. Serotyping by micro-immunofluorescence can differentiate LGV from non-LGV strains. To date, there have been no studies using Nucleic Acid Amplification Techniques (NAAT) and the best method of detection may be by culture, since the former may be insensitive because of inhibitors.

REITER'S SYNDROME

Reiter's syndrome is defined by the American College of Rheumatology as "an episode of peripheral arthritis of more than one month duration occurring in association with urethritis and/or cervicitis"[12]. A classic presentation of reactive arthritis accompanied by urogenital, mucocutaneous and ocular inflammation is unusual, and *"formes fruste"* are common. The syndrome is often mis-diagnosed as one of the other sero-negative spondylo-arthropathies such as psoriatic arthritis, ankylosing sponylitis or the arthritis of inflammatory bowel disease. This makes accurate epidemiological data difficult to compile.

The syndrome exists both as a sexually acquired reactive arthrosis (SARA) and a less common epidemic dysenteric form, the latter having been associated with *Shigella flexnerii, Salmonella* spp, *Yersinia enterocolitica* and *Campylobacter jejuni* but *Shigella soneii* is apparently devoid of this complication.

Peak onset is in the third decade but it may appear in children and the elderly. Incidence is probably around 33 per 100,000 in males[13].

SARA affects men more often than it does women. The male to female ratio was thought to be 20:1 but this was the result of under reporting in women (where cervicitis and less severe disease went unrecognised) and observations in cohorts from predominately male populations. Male to female ratios range from 9:1 to 5:1.

The disease is a symptom complex which may be straightforward to diagnose but fewer than one third present with all definite systems involved. A good sexual history therefore is an important aid to diagnosis.

Urethritis is an early symptom, occurring 2-4 weeks after sexual exposure or diarrhoeal illness. Men may have prostatitis and women cervicitis or vaginitis. These symptoms can also occur in patients with the post dysenteric form.

Ocular findings are seen in 50% of the sexually acquired form and 75% of the dysenteric. Conjunctivitis is common with keratitis, iritis and uveitis less so. All of these may be recurrent.

Arthritis is usually the last clinical feature to appear being polyarticular and asymetric with effusions. Any joint can be involved but favoured sites are the ankles, knees and toes with later involvement including fingers and wrists. 50% of patients have sacroiliitis and axial spine involvement. Inflammation of the bony insertion of tendons and ligaments is found in some patients, particularly affecting the Achilles tendon and plantar fascia. Dactylitis can produce sausage shaped fingers or toes.

Dermatological involvement is seen in approximately half of cases with painless, shallow ulcerations on the lips, palate and tongue with circinate balanitis a common feature. Keratodermia blennorrhagica is seen on the soles of the feet or palms of the hands as erythematous macules which form hyper-keratotic papules.

Unusual complications include cardiac conduction abnormalities, myocarditis, aortitis and neurological findings such as hemiplegia and peripheral neuropathy.

Laboratory findings are generally non-specific and unhelpful with raised C-reactive protein levels and erythrocyte sedimentation rate. Mild anaemia and leucocytocis (with a shift to the left) can be found.

Joint fluid may reveal a polymorphonucler lymphocytocis and elevated protein. A Gram stain should be negative for organisms.

C. trachomatis is obviously not the only trigger infection to produce the syndrome but researchers have shown some association. Elementary bodies in joint fluid and synovial biopsies of patients with Reiter's syndrome have been demonstrated[14]. Both PCR and LCR have been used more recently to demonstrate the presence of the organism in stored synovial samples[15] and synovial fluid samples[16].

SOME FURTHER CONSIDERATIONS

As can be seen from the above Chlamydia presents a real and increasing danger to the general psychological and sexual health of men. This is not only because of its incidence and clinical manifestations, but also from the fact that it is often sub-clinical, with patient and health provider insufficiently aware of the likelihood of its presence.

The situation may be improved by two developments. Firstly, advances in the technology of detection should make testing less invasive, and therefore more acceptable. This should also facilitate the second development, which is screening. Screening should reveal more of the endemic infection present in both the male and female population and thereby reduce not only the numbers of complications arising from infection but also background prevalence.

A note of caution, however, should be raised here. Women have traditionally been seen as the ideal (i.e. easiest) population to screen since they access health care in appropriate locations where detection can be employed. GU Medicine, Family Planning, Antenatal and Well Women Clinics are locations where sexually active women can be found and screening applied. With men the situation is quite different, especially for the young. There exists no focus of health care where men can be found *en-masse* and therefore, innovative approaches must be sought. These might include screening at social functions (e.g. music events and youth centres) or even schools or institutions of higher education. In this way men may be brought into screening.

Until they are, the temptation is to screen the easy target i.e. women, but this only addresses half of the problem. It could allow men to permit the responsibility for good sexual health to rest with their female partners. Men may thus be disenfranchised and come to regard Chlamydia in the same way some of them presently consider other issues of sexual health e.g. contraception and termination of pregnancy, as the responsibility of women.

Non-invasive screening techniques for Chlamydia combined with appropriate educational interventions which raise awareness could make men sexually healthier in the more holistic sense.

REFERENCES

1. Parkes KS, Dickson PB, Richie CM. (1997). Spontaneous Clearance of *Chlamydia trachomatis* Infection in Untreated Patients *Sex Trans Dis* **24**(4):229–35.
2. Cohen DA, Nsuami M, Martin DH, *et al.* (1999). Repeated School Based Screening for Sexually Transmitted Diseases: A Feasible Strategy for Reaching Adolescents. *Paediatrics* **104**(6): 1281–1285.
3. Jebakumar SPR, Storey C, Lusher M *et al.* (1995). Value of screening for oro-pharyngeal *Chlamydia trachomatis* infection.*J Clin Path* **48:** 658–61.
4. Quinn TC, Goodell SE, McKritchian E, *et al.* (1981). *Chlamydia trachomatis* Proctitis. *N Eng J Med* **305:** 195–200.
5. Hori S, Tsutsumi Y. (1995). Histological Differentiation between Chlamydial and Bacterial Epididymitis: non-destructive and proliferative *vs.* destructive and abscess-forming – immunohistochemical and clinicopathological findings *Human Pathology* **26**(4): 402–7.

6. Krieger JN, Jacobs R, Ross SO. (2000). Detecting Urethral and Prostatic Inflammation in Patients with Chronic Prostatitis. *Urology* **55**(2): 186–192.
7. Ballard RC, Koornhof HJ, Mausenbaum E, *et al.* The Role of *Chlamydia trachomatis* in the Aetiology of Chronic Prostatitis and Treatment of the Condition with Azithromycin. 12th International Congress of Chemotherapy. Florence 1981 Abstract 233.
8. Bruce A W, Reid G. (1989). Prostatitis Associated with *Chlamydia trachomatis* in 6 Patients. *J Urol* **142**: 1006–7.
9. Poletti F, Medici MC, Alinovi A *et al.* (1985). Isolation of *Chlamydia trachomatis* from the prostate cells in patients affected by acute abacterial prostatitis. *J Urol* **134**: 691–3.
10. Doble A, Thomas BJ, Walker MM, *et al.* (1989). The Role of *Chlamydia trachomatis* in Chronic Abacterial Prostatitis: A Study Using Ultrasound Guided Biopsy. *J Urol* **141**: 332–3.
11. Krüger JN, Riley DE, Roberts MC *et al.* (1996). Prokaryotic DNA sequences in patients with chronic idiopathic prostatitis. *J Clin Microbiol* **34**: 3120–8.
12. Willkens RF, Arnett FC, Bitter T, *et al.* (1981). Reiter's Syndrome: Evaluation of Preliminary Criteria for Definite Disease. *Arthritis and Rheum* **24**(6): 844–9.
13. Cush JJ, Lipsky PE. (1993). Reiter's Syndrome and Reactive Arthritis in Arthritis and Allied Conditions: McCarty D J, Koopman W J, eds. 12th Edition Philadelphia: Lea and Febiger: **106**, 1–78.
14. Keat, Thomas D, Dixey J. (1987). *Chlamydia trachomatis* and reactive arthritis: the missing link *Lancet* **1**: 72–74.
15. Taylor-Robinson D, Gilroy CB, Thomas BJ. (1992). Detection of *Chlamydia trachomatis* DNA in joints of reactive arthritis patients by Polymerase Chain Reaction. *Lancet* **340**: 81–82.
16. Nikkari S, Puolakkainen M, Yli-Kerttula U *et al.* (1997). Ligase chain reaction in detection of chlamydial DNA in synovial fluid cells *Br J Rheumat* **36**: 763–5.

SUGGESTED FURTHER READING

Centers for Disease Control and Prevention (1993). Recommendation for the prevention and management of Chlamydia trachomatis infections *Morbid. Mortal. Weekly Report;* **42** (RR-12): 1–39.

Stamm WE, Holmes KK. (1990).Chlamydia trachomatis infections of the adult.Sexually Transmitted Diseases: Eds: Holmes K K, Mårdh P-A, Sparling P F, Wiesner P G New York: Mc Graw Hill; New York: 181–194.

Herbner TD. (1996). Ultrasound in the Assessment of the Acute Scrotum. *J Clin Ultrasound* **24**(8): 405–21.

Purvis K, Christiansen E. (1996). The Impact of Infection on Sperm Quality in Human Reproduction **11**: 2 Suppl; 31–41.

Hughes RA, Keat AC. (1994). Reiter's Syndrome and Reactive Arthritis: A Current Review. Seminars in Arthritis & Rheumatism. **24**(3): 190–210.

CHAPTER 8

Complications in the female and their management

Karen E Rogstad

Department of Genitourinary Medicine,
Royal Hallamshire Hospital, Sheffield, UK

Chlamydia trachomatis infection of the female genital tract can vary from an asymptomatic self-limiting infection to a severe debilitating illness with serious long-term complications both of the reproductive tract itself and also as a more disseminated disease. Whilst in the asymptomatic phase, ongoing damage to the fallopian tubes may be occurring and the diagnosis may only be made many years later, when complications are detected.

Initial entry to the body usually occurs through penetrative sexual intercourse, with organisms being deposited in the urethra, vagina and endocervix. Ascending infection then occurs, via the uterus, to the fallopian tubes to cause silent or overt pelvic inflammatory disease (PID), with resultant complications. Dissemination may then progress to the liver. Autoimmune responses to the bacteria complicate the picture resulting in worsening of PID or a reactive arthritis. Potential complications are shown in **Table 1** and illustrated in **Figure 1**.

Direct or auto-inoculation results in conjunctivitis, and anal sexual intercourse can result in a proctitis although this appears to be rare in women. Similarly, pharyngitis in women is unusual. If present in a pregnant woman, Chlamydia can result in neonatal infection and post-partum complications in the mother.

Symptoms may appear soon after infection, or many months later and untreated latent infection may be reactivated at a later date.

Table 1. Complications of *Chlamydia trachomatis* in women

Site		symptoms, signs and complications
Urethra	urethritis	frequency/dysuria
Cervix	cervicitis	mucopurulent vaginal discharge
Uterus	endometritis	vaginal discharge irregular bleeding post coital bleeding
Fallopian tubes	salpingitis	pelvic inflammatory disease ectopic pregnancy tubal infertility chronic pelvic pain
Liver	perihepatitis	right upper quadrant pain
Bartholins gland	bartholinitis	swelling and pain of vulva
Conjunctiva	conjunctivitis	discharge from eye
Systemic	Reiter's syndrome	arthritis (large joints) iritis keratodermia blenorrhagica
Pregnancy/Neonate	pneumonitis conjunctivitis post-partum endometritis	

PATHOPHYSIOLOGY

C. trachomatis enters into columnar or transitional epithelial cells of the genital tract, rectum and peritoneum. The reticulate body of the Chlamydia replicates and, when new elementary bodies are assembled, they leave the cell, with resultant cell death. In the fallopian tube, there is subepithelial inflammation, epithelial ulceration and scarring. Damage is mediated by the cell death and exacerbated by a delayed hypersensitivity reaction to chlamydial 60kDa heat shock proteins (HSP-60).

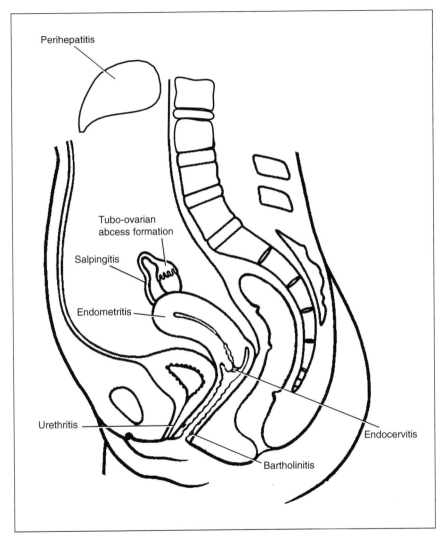

Figure 1. Sites of infection with *Chlamydia trachomatis*.

ACUTE URETHRAL SYNDROME

This develops as a result of urethral infection, although the majority of women with chlamydial infection of this site are asymptomatic

The diagnosis should be considered in women presenting with symptoms of cystitis, particularly where the dysuria has been present for more than one week. Examination may reveal meatal discharge, erythema or swelling but is usually normal. A clue to a urethral rather than bladder cause for the symptoms is suggested by lack of suprapubic tenderness, absence of haematuria and a urethral smear showing more than 10 polymorphs per high power field. A mid-stream urine specimen will reveal a culture negative pyuria.

CERVICITIS

Women with cervicitis can be asymptomatic or complain of vaginal discharge, which may be yellow or green. If there is coexistent bacterial vaginosis (BV) (which is often the case) then they may also complain of odour. Post-coital bleeding occurs in some.

The cervix may appear completely normal despite being infected with Chlamydia. However, at least a third may show evidence of infection with either a hypertrophic ectopy of the endocervix, as manifested by cervical oedema, congestion and bleeding (19%), or have a mucopurulent discharge (37%)[1].

A cotton tipped swab inserted into the endocervix detects mucopus in the presence of a mucopurulent chlamydial cervicitis. Contact bleeding, on taking swabs or when performing cervical cytology, is also suggestive of chlamydial infection.

Cervicitis can also be diagnosed by microscopy of an endocervical swab, with a finding of more than 30 polymorphonuclear leucocytes (PMNs) per x 1000 field suggesting a diagnosis of Chlamydia or gonorrhoea. However, the diagnosis of Chlamydia itself requires specific testing and is discussed elsewhere. The inflammatory response associated with chlamydial cervicitis can obscure the endocervical cells on PAP smears, resulting in inadequate cervical cytology. Any woman who has a smear reported as "inflammatory changes" requires testing for the detection of *C. trachomatis*.

Although there is an increased prevalence of *C. trachomatis* in those with cervical ectopy the reason for this is unclear. It may be either because the organism itself causes ectopy, because those with ectopy are predisposed to acquiring Chlamydia, or ectopy of the cervix in women increases shedding of the organism.

ENDOMETRITIS

Nearly half of patients with chlamydial cervicitis will also have an endometritis. This can be asymptomatic or the patient may complain of menorrhagia, metrorrhagia or post-coital bleeding. Endometrial biopsy shows plasma cells in the stroma and polymorphonuclear leucocytes in the superficial epithelium, but is rarely undertaken. Culture or EIA tests for CT from the endocervix may be negative. It is to be hoped that newer DNA amplification methods will aid diagnosis.

PELVIC INFLAMMATORY DISEASE

Pelvic inflammatory disease (PID) occurs when there is upper genital tract infection and can be used to refer to salpingitis alone or include endometritis. It can be acute, sub-acute, chronic or silent. Up to 80% of cases of acute PID in the developed world are due to a sexually transmitted infection, and European studies suggest CT is the cause of at least 60% of cases. Accurate diagnosis is difficult without the use of invasive techniques such as laparoscopy therefore data on frequency are difficult to interpret. However it appears that between 10 and 40% of women infected with *C. trachomatis* develop PID[2]. There is often co-infection with BV associated organisms and *Neisseria gonorrhoeae* may also be present.

The incidence is greatest in 15-19 year olds, and the relative risk of acquiring PID in women is also highest in this group. The combined oral contraceptive pill confers some protection against ascending infection, and if PID does occur it is usually less severe. The risk of CT causing PID is increased by the presence of an intrauterine contraceptive device (IUCD), particularly at initial insertion or when it is changed. Certain types of IUCD e.g. those with progesterone appear to pose less risk than other types. The risk of CT causing salpingitis is also increased by manipulation of the cervix during termination of pregnancy or other gynaecological procedures.

Recurrences of PID are frequent and can be due to Chlamydia persistence because of incomplete treatment, re-infection as a result of failure to perform partner notification or a new infected partner. Recurrences also occur as an ascending infection of other bacteria from the lower genital tract into the already damaged fallopian tubes.

PID presents as acute lower abdominal or pelvic pain. There may be deep dyspareunia, vaginal bleeding and discharge as well as pyrexia. Clinical examination can reveal lower abdominal tenderness, adnexal tenderness and cervical excitation (pain on cervical movement). Bilateral masses may be felt, particularly if there is tubo-ovarian abcess formation. In some, investigations show a raised white cell count and ESR. However, in silent chlamydial PID no symptoms or signs may be present although ongoing tubal damage is occurring. Previous tubal ligation does not exclude the diagnosis as was previously thought[3].

The gold standard for diagnosis has been laparoscopy but this will fail to detect milder cases. Similarly, endometrial biopsy may be helpful but can be negative. Neither investigation is usually needed.

The management of PID is described in chapter 5 and consists of oral or intravenous antibiotics active against *C. trachomatis*, combined with metronidazole to cover anaerobes which are also usually present. The presence of tubo-ovarian abcesses may require surgical intervention.

Physicians should have a low threshold for diagnosis and initiation of therapy particularly in adolescents, as even a 3-day delay in treatment can cause a threefold increase in risk of infertility[4]. It is therefore recommended that any sexually active adolescent presenting with lower abdominal pain with adnexal and cervical motion tenderness should receive treatment if no other cause is identified[5].

Whenever a diagnosis of PID is made, pregnancy testing should be performed as recent data has shown that ectopic pregnancy may be an acute as well as a long-term complication of chlamydial infection .

COMPLICATIONS OF CHLAMYDIAL PELVIC INFLAMMATORY DISEASE

As PID worsens, tubo-ovarian abcesses can form and peritonitis develop, as well as Fitz-Hugh-Curtis syndrome. Long-term complications of PID include ectopic pregnancy, tubal infertility and chronic pelvic pain. The risk of sequaele increases disproportionately with subsequent infections. For ectopic pregnancy or tubal infertility the odds ratio increases from 6 after one episode of PID to 17 after two episodes[6].

An ectopic pregnancy is life threatening, resulting in 10% of deaths in England that occur as a complication of pregnancy, childbirth or the puerperium. In women who have had PID the risk of ectopic pregnancy is increased by 7-10 times, and 43% of cases of ectopic pregnancy may be due to Chlamydia, either recognised or unrecognised[7]. Recent evidence from Sweden suggests that ectopic pregnancy may be an acute, as well as, long-term complication of infection with *C. trachomatis*. Researchers found a strong correlation between ectopic pregnancy rates and rate of chlamydial infection in the same year for women 20-24 years of age[8].

As well as causing ectopic pregnancy, the tubal damage which occurs as a result of tubal inflammation, scarring and subsequent occlusion can result in primary or secondary infertility. It is estimated that 50% of cases of infertility are due to tubal factors of which 50% of these are caused by *C. trachomatis*, and many give no history of previous PID[9].

Chronic pelvic pain occurs in more than 15% of women with previous episodes of PID, increasing from an incidence of 11% after one episode to 66% after 3 or more episodes. It appears to be correlated with the presence of peritoneal adhesions.

BARTHOLINITIS

The Bartholins ducts open into the posterior third of the labia minora, and although infection with subsequent abscess formation is more usually associated with gonococcal infections, Bartholinitis can also be caused by Chlamydia. It typically presents with local pain and swelling and examination reveals a tender abscess of the lower labia, which may be fluctuant.

Management is by antibiotic therapy but surgical treatment with marsupialization may be necessary.

FITZ-HUGH-CURTIS SYNDROME

The term Fitz-Hugh-Curtis Syndrome (FHC) is used for the perihepatitis associated with genital chlamydial or gonococcal infection. Although first described in the latter it is more frequently associated with Chlamydia. There is an acute inflammatory reaction on the liver capsule and adjacent peritoneum, but there is no involvement of the liver parenchyma. *C. trachomatis* organisms can sometimes be isolated from the hepatic surface. This condition occurs in 5-15% of women with laparoscopically diagnosed salpingitis and symptoms suggestive of it are found in 20%. It may result from direct spread of Chlamydia from the fallopian tubes via the peritoneum. However it is likely that spread through the lymphatic system and haematogenous spread may also occur, as it has been found in women who have had tubal ligation and also rarely in men with gonococcal urethritis. Evidence suggests an association with previous chlamydial infection, as titres of antibody to CT are significantly higher in those with the syndrome compared to those women with CT PID and no perihepatitis. Patients with FHC also have high titres of antibodies to chlamydial 60kDa heat shock protein.

Patients present with right, upper quadrant pain which may occur alone or with symptoms of vaginal discharge or PID. Fever, nausea and vomiting may be present. The pain can be pleuritic and there may be referred pain to the shoulder and back. Symptoms can be exacerbated by breathing, coughing and movement. The upper abdominal pain can precede the pelvic pain by several days and may be so severe that the PID symptoms are ignored. On examination, there is tenderness under the right costal margin and a rub may be present in severe cases. Signs of general peritonitis can occur. White cell count and ESR are raised in approximately 30% and mild bilirubin and liver enzyme increases are found in less than 50%. Chest X-ray may show pleural fluid. Diagnosis is usually based on clinical suspicion, in the presence of a normal ultrasound of the gallbladder and common bile ducts.

A definitive diagnosis is made by laparoscopy when purulent fibrinous peritonitis of the liver capsule is found. Adhesions between the liver and abdominal wall can occur and typical thin, avascular "violin-string" adhesions may be found in more advanced cases.

PREGNANCY AND THE NEONATE

There is little and conflicting evidence to implicate CT in chorioamnionitis and adverse pregnancy outcome. DNA amplification has found it to be present in the amniotic fluid of 6.7% of women with pre-labour amniorrhexis but the significance of this is not known[10]. However late post partum endometritis is well recognised and occurs in 30% of women with antenatal CT infection. On examination there may be mild uterine tenderness, or the patient may be asymptomatic, and if unrecognised and untreated secondary infertility may result.

Infants of mothers with chlamydial infection will develop conjunctivitis in 18-50% of cases and pneumonia in 11-20%. Although these are thought to result from contact with infected vaginal secretions, there have been cases reported where neonatal chlamydial infection was found in infants delivered by caesarean section in the presence of intact membranes[11]. Chlamydial conjunctivitis presents 5-10 days after delivery whereas pneumonitis usually presents at 2-3 weeks. Rarely there may be severe respiratory failure, and there is some evidence to suggest long-term respiratory disease may result[12,13]. Whether serous otitis media, small for dates babies and failure to thrive in infancy occur secondary to vertically acquired Chlamydia is controversial.

REACTIVE ARTHRITIS

This term replaces the former term of Reiter's Syndrome which, by definition, requires the presence of conjunctivitis, arthritis and urethritis, thus contributing to the high male:female ratio. Viable Chlamydiae have now been found in synovium and synovial fluid using nucleic acid amplification techniques. It is thought the Chlamydiae are transported from the genital tract in macrophages or dendritic cells and that hypersensitivity to chlamydial HSP 60, as in PID, may play a role[14]. The presence of HLA-B27 appears to increase susceptibility, severity and persistence. There is an association with the other spondyloarthropathies.

The arthritis typically affects large weight-bearing joints and occurs several weeks after infection. There may also be iritis, conjunctivitis and keratodermia blenorrhagica (circinate balanitis is an associated feature in male cases).

Management is of the underlying chlamydial infection, non-steroidal anti-inflammatory drugs and physiotherapy. Bed rest may be appropriate in the early stages. One trial has shown possible benefit of long-term tetracycline[15] and results of a further trial using azithromycin are awaited.

OTHER COMPLICATIONS

Although there have been occasional case reports of pneumonitis in immunocompetent adults, there is no real evidence. There have been some suggestions that genital *C. trachomatis* may be implicated in culture-negative endocervicitis, meningo-encephalitis, peritonitis and post-menopausal vaginitis.

The early diagnosis and management of chlamydial infection of the female genital tract is essential to protect the reproductive health of women. In the absence of a national screening programme every doctor and nurse must consider chlamydial infection a possibility in any sexually active girl or woman, and in neonates with respiratory or conjunctival problems. Only by doing so will women and babies be protected from the debilitating acute and long-term sequelae of this disease.

Acknowledgements
I would like to thank Chris Taylor for secretarial support and Martin Talbot for advice on the manuscript.

REFERENCES

1. Harrison HR *et al.* (1985). Cervical *Chlamydia trachomatis* infection in university women: Relationship to history, contraception, ectopy and cervicitis. *Am J Obstet Gynaecol* **153:** 241–4.
2. Stum W, Guinan M, Johsac *et al.* (1984). Effects of treatment regimes for *N. gonorrhoea* on simultaneous infection with *Chlamydia trachomatis*. *N Engl J Med* **310:** 545–9.
3. Leugur M, Duvivier R. (2000). Pelvic inflammatory disease after tubal sterilization: a review. *Obstetrical & Gynaecological Survey* **55:** 41–50.
4. Hillis S, Jeosoef R, Marcbanks P *et al.* (1993). Delayed care of pelvic inflammatory disease as a risk factor for impaired fertility *Am J Obstet Gynaecol* **168:** 1503–9.
5. Centres for Disease Control and Prevention: 1998 Guidelines for treatment of sexually transmitted diseases. *MMWR Mrb Mortal Wkly Rep 47(RR-1)*; **1:** 1-118, 1998.
6. Westrom C. (1994). Sexually transmitted diseases and infertility *Sex Trans Dis* **21:** 532–37.
7. Sexually transmitted diseases quarterly report: genital chlamydial infection, ectopic pregnancy and syphilis in England and Wales. (2000). *Commun Dis Rep CDR wkly* **10:** 116–117.
8. Egger M, Low N, Smith GD, Lindblon B, Hermann B. (1998). Screening for chlamydial infection and the risk of ectopic pregnancy in a county in Sweden: ecological analysis. *Br Med J* **316:** 1776–80
9. World Health Organization Task Force on the prevention and management of infertility Tubal Infertility: Serologic Relationship to Post Chlamydial and Gonococcal Infection (1995). *Sex Trans Dis* **22:** 71–77.
10. Ville Y, Carroll SG, Watts P *et al.*(1997). *Chlamydia trachomatis* infection in pre-labour amniorrhexis *Br J Obstet Gynaecol* **104:** 1091–1093.
11. Ratelle S, Keno D, Hardwood M, Etkind PH. (1997). Neonatal Chlamydial infections in Massachusetts 1992-1993, *Am J Prev Med* **13:** 221–224.
12. Harrison HR, Phil D, Taussig LM *et al.* (1982). *Chlamydia trachomatis* and chronic respiratory diseases in childhood *Pediatr Inf Dis* **1:** 29–33.
13. Weiss SG, Newcomb RW, Beem MJ. (1986). Pulmonary assessment of children after chlamydial pneumonia of infancy *J Paediatr* **108:** 659–64.
14. Gaston JSH. (2000). Immunological basis of chlamydia induced reactive arthritis *Sex Trans Infects* **76:** 15: 6–161.
15. Lauhio A, Leirisalo Repo M, Lahdevirta J *et al.* (1991). Double-blind, placebo – controlled study of three-month treatment with lymecycline in reactive arthritis with special reference to Chlamydia arthritis. *Arthritis Rheum* **34:** 6–14.

BIBLIOGRAPHY

Holmes KK, Sparling PF, Mårdh P-A *et al.* (1999). Sexually Transmitted Diseases 3rd edition, McGraw – Hill. ISBN 0-07-029688-X

Chlamydia trachomatis *infection in fallopian tube disease – the Swedish experience*

Per-Anders Mårdh
Department of Obstetrics and Gynaecology,
University Hospital, Lund, Sweden

INTRODUCTION

The Swedish effort to reduce the pool of carriers of *Chlamydia trachomatis* is a textbook example of a highly successful public health intervention programme to reduce a disease and thereby also its sequelae. Thus the intensive screening programme of the agent performed on a national basis resulted in a massive reduction of pelvic inflammatory disease (PID) and also of chlamydial infections in the newborn, e.g. of eye and lung infections. The efforts are also likely to have reduced late sequelae, e.g. of asthma, obstructive lung disease, as well as of infertility, ectopic pregnancy and chronic abdominal pain. The present study reviews the initial Swedish Chlamydia research and the national public health efforts regarding screening and counselling activities in the field.

HOW DID IT ALL START?

After a visit to Seattle and contact with Dr Say-Ping Wang, the author, and later also the author's PhD students, started research into how to simplify the diagnosis of chlamydial infections. When this research became fruitful we started to study the local epidemiology of genital *C. trachomatis* infections. In 1975, at a meeting in Lake Placid, US, we were able to present a method that meant a breakthrough in the diagnosis of infections by *C. trachomatis*, i.e. the use of cycloheximide-treated McCoy cell cultures[1]. At the same meeting, we presented evidence for *C. trachomatis* being an etiological agent of PID[2]. In 1977, we published a study confirming such an etiological relationship[3].

By the end of 1976, we offered the possibility for routine diagnosis of *C. trachomatis* for our laboratory's catchment area. We carried out routine testing of women attending the outpatient department of Obstetrics and Gynaecology at Lund University Hospital, as well as women hospitalised at the clinic. These studies confirmed that genital chlamydial infections were common in these cohorts. Thus, 25% of all women with vaginal discharge at that time had a genital chlamydial infection[4]. Of those with gonorrhoea, one in four also had an infection by *C. trachomatis*. The opposite was also true. Partner notification detected a chlamydial infection in more than half of the sexual contacts to an index case[5].

EVIDENCE OF CORRELATION BETWEEN PID AND GENITAL CHLAMYDIAL INFECTION

In any study of salpingitis, it is essential that the diagnosis is correctly confirmed. So far, laparoscopy/laparatomy have ranked highest in accuracy among diagnostic methods[6]. In laparoscopically confirmed cases of salpingitis, samples that we collected from the fallopian tubes revealed the presence of *C. trachomatis* by the use of tissue cell cultures[3,7]. In such cases, we also found a significant antibody response to the agent[7,8]. Also histological findings supported a causal relationship[9]. In animal models, e.g. in grivet monkeys, *C. trachomatis* provoked salpingitis[10,11].

We presented data supporting a canalicular spread of Chlamydia organisms to the tubes by showing evidence of endometritis in PID cases being caused by *C. trachomatis*[12], where histological sections showed a characteristic plasma cell infiltration.

In women with chronic abdominal pain[13] and in those with involuntary childlessness[14], there is evidence of a past infection with *C. trachomatis*. We also found evidence of complications of PID being due to an agent, as in periappendicitis[15], perihepatitis[16-18], peritonitis, perisplenitis and perisigmoiditis as a consequence of chlamydial infection spreading from the tubes to the abdominal cavity.

Use of oral contraceptives may modulate the course of PID and therefore also the rate of sequelae of chlamydial salpingitis[19,20]. We found that perihepatitis was a rather uncommon complication in Chlamydia PID cases in women on the pill, but rather common in such cases *not* taking the pill.

POSITIVE IMPACT ON PUBLIC HEALTH BY SCREENING FOR *C. TRACHOMATIS*

Knowledge of a high prevalence of genital chlamydial infections in the general Swedish population at the beginning of the 1980s led to the start of an impressive national screening programme for *C. trachomatis*. For some years during the mid-1980s the number of Chlamydia samples collected exceeded half a million (the Swedish population at that time was approx. 8.5 million). The outcome of the programme was a marked drop over the next few years in the number of diagnosed PID cases[21] and some years later of ectopic pregnancy cases[22].

There was a simultaneous drop in the number of chlamydial infections and of gonorrhoea cases after diagnostic possibilities of the former were established. The reduction of both these infections started some years before similar trends were seen in other countries. It should be noted that tests for *C. trachomatis* and *Neisseria gonorrhoea* were generally done simultaneously in the Swedish screening programmes. A tetracycline (often doxycycline or lymecycline) was the drug generally chosen to treat chlamydial infections in Sweden; a therapy which at that time was also curative for the vast majority of gonorrhoea infections. Thus screening for genital chlamydial infections also meant a concomitant decrease in the carrier rate of gonococci in the general population. This contributed to a decrease in the rate of gonococcal salpingitis and its complications and sequelae.

The rate of ectopic pregnancy in Sweden decreased in parallel with that of PID, but with some years delay. In a group of Swedish women, a mean time lag of 7.5 years was found between a diagnosed episode of PID and that of ectopic pregnancy. The time delay may partly reflect the trend among Swedish women to wish to conceive at a much later age than when they generally contract their first chlamydial infection.

There is evidence that a genital chlamydial infection may induce hypersensitivity reactions, (*via* similarities between human and chlamydial heat shock proteins [HSP-60]), that can interfere with the ability to conceive and also contribute to failure of *in vitro* fertilisation (IVF) attempts[23].

As a consequence of the wide spread of genital chlamydial infection in young Swedes, "youth clinics" were opened in many Swedish cities. Teenagers can attend these clinics, without pre-booking consultation time. At the clinics the teenagers meet midwives, who are supported by gynaecologists if necessary. The midwives often gain the teenager's confidence, so that counselling in risk reduction is very successful. Contraceptive advice also plays a central role in the youth clinic programme; the clinics were also intended to try to reduce teenage pregnancies.

MOTIVATIONS FOR SCREENING PREGNANT WOMEN

We found evidence of intrauterine infections by *C. trachomatis*, i.e. in cases of Premature Rupture of Membranes (PROM)[24] and we demonstrated serological evidence of a past *C. trachomatis* infection in many cases of ectopic pregnancy[25].

There is new evidence that *C. trachomatis* may also play an important role in premature birth in women who have an intrauterine infection by the agent.[26] Thus up to 10% of children born prematurely may be already infected *in utero*, as evidenced by tests of cord blood for antichlamydia IgM antibodies.

We and other Swedish researchers also reported on evidence of pelvic chlamydial infection after elective abortion performed within 14th week of gestation[27,28]. In the later study, positive *C. trachomatis* cervical cultures supported a causal relationship.

INFECTIONS IN NEWBORNS

Transfer of *C. trachomatis* at delivery from an infected mother to the offspring may cause pneumonia in infants. The pneumonia often presents several weeks after delivery when the child has developed the capability to react with delayed hypersensitivity reactions to the agent[29]. It is notable that newborns are often transiently colonised in the eyes by *C. trachomatis*[30], but will never develop any signs of infection.

CHOICE OF THERAPEUTIC AGENT IN PREGNANT WOMEN

Therapy of genital chlamydial infections in pregnant women is restricted to the choice of a tetracycline (often doxycycline), erythromycin or azithromycin. In a study comparing Tetralysal® and Azithromax®, we found no difference in their efficiency to cure genital chlamydial infections in females, as evidenced from negative post-therapy cultures of *C. trachomatis*[31].

We also stressed the importance of early partner notification in any therapy of an index case infected by *C. trachomatis*[5].

As the infection in the pregnant woman may have been contracted before she conceived, the infection has had the chance to ascend to the uterine mucosa. Thus pregnant women should be treated as if they have a PID (even if the Chlamydia diagnosis is only based on a positive test from the lower genital tract or by analysis of voided urine samples).

COST ESTIMATES OF GENITAL CHLAMYDIAL INFECTION

Cost estimates of screening programmes for genital chlamydial infections have shown that they (on a local or national level) are cost-effective if the carrier rate in the population is 6%[32,33], if one does not include an assumed percentage of clinical silent PID. When including a percentage of such cases, other workers found screening programmes to be cost-effective at a carrier rate of only 3%. However, all cost estimates presented so far have never considered the enormous costs of life-long sequelae, e.g. of obstructive lung disease, in persons infected at delivery by a Chlamydia-infected mother. Other costs seldom considered are those related to giving birth to premature born twins after IVF (motivated by a previous chlamydial infection that had resulted in tubal occlusion). Thus to be realistic, any cost estimates should also include life-long sequelae in persons prematurely born, as a consequence of a chlamydial infection in his/her mother.

REFERENCES

1. Ripa T, Mårdh P-A. (1977). A new simplified culture technique for *Chlamydia trachomatis*. In: Holmes KK, Hobson D, eds. Non-gonococcal Urethritis and Related Infections. Washington DC: *Am Soc Microbiol* 32–37.
2. Mårdh P-A, Ripa KT, Wang S-P, Weström L. (1977). *Chlamydia trachomatis* as an aetiological agent in acute salpingitis. In: Holmes KK, Hobson D, eds. Non-gonococcal Urethritis and Related Infections. Washington DC: *Am Soc Microbiol* 77–83.
3. Mårdh P-A, Ripa KT, Svensson L, Weström L. (1977). *Chlamydia trachomatis* infection in patients with acute salpingitis. *N Engl J Med* **23:** 1377–9.
4. Svensson L, Weström L, Mårdh P-A. (1981). *Chlamydia trachomatis* in women attending a gynaecological outpatient clinic with lower genital tract infection. *Br J Vener Dis* **57:** 259–62.
5. Thelin I, Wennström A-M, Mårdh P-A. (1980). Contact tracing in patients with genital chlamydial infection. *Br J Vener Dis* **56:** 259–62.
6. Weström L, Mårdh P-A. Salpingitis. In: Holmes KK, Mårdh P-A, Sparling F, Wiesner P, eds. Sexually Transmitted Diseases. New York: McGraw-Hill, 1984: 615–63.
7. Svensson L, Weström L, Mårdh P-A. (1981). Acute salpingitis with *Chlamydia trachomatis* isolated from the fallopian tubes: clinical, cultural and serological findings. *Sex Trans Dis* **8:** 51–5.
8. Treharne JD, Ripa KT, Mårdh P-A, Svensson L, Weström L, Darougar S. (1979). Antibodies to *Chlamydia trachomatis* in acute salpingitis. *Br J Vener Dis* **55:** 26–9.
9. Möller BR, Weström L, Ahrons S, Ripa KT, Svensson L, von Mecklenburg C, Henrikson H, Mårdh P-A. (1979). *Chlamydia trachomatis* infection of the Fallopian tubes. Histological finding in two patients. *Br J Vener Dis* **55:** 422–8.
10. Möller BR, Freundt EA, Mårdh P-A. (1980). Experimental pelvic inflammatory disease provoked by *Chlamydia trachomatis* and *Mycoplasma hominis* in grivet monkeys. *Am J Obstet Gynecol* **138** Suppl: 1017–21.
11. Möller BR, Mårdh P-A. (1980). Experimental salpingitis in grivet monkeys by *Chlamydia trachomatis*. Modes of spread of infection to the Fallopian tubes. *Acta Path Microbiol Scand* **88B:** 107–14.

12. Mårdh P-A, Möller BR, Ingerslev HJ, Nüssler E, Weström L, Wölner-Hanssen P. (1981). Endometritis caused by *Chlamydia trachomatis*. *Br J Vener Dis* **57:** 191–5.
13. Wölner-Hanssen P, Mårdh P-A, Weström L, Svensson L. (1983). Laparoscopy in women with chlamydial infection and pelvic pain. A comparison of patients with and without salpingitis. *Obst Gynecol* **61:** 299–303.
14. Svensson L, Mårdh P-A, Weström L. (1983). Infertility after acute salpingitis with special reference to *Chlamydia trachomatis*. *Steril Fertil* **40:** 322–9.
15. Mårdh P-A, Wølner-Hanssen P. (1985). Periappendicitis and chlamydial salpingitis. *Surg Gynecol Obstet* **160:** 304–6.
16. Wølner-Hanssen P, Weström L, Mårdh P-A. (1980). Perihepatitis and chlamydial salpingitis. *Lancet* **i:** 901–4.
17. Wølner-Hanssen P, Weström L, Mårdh P-A. (1981). Perihepatitis and chlamydial salpingitis. *Obst Gyn Survey* **36:** 44–5.
18. Wølner-Hanssen P, Svensson L, Weström L, Mårdh P-A. (1982). Isolation of *Chlamydia trachomatis* from the liver capsule in Fitz-Hugh-Curtis syndrome. *New Engl J Med* **306:** 113.
19. Svensson L, Mårdh P-A, Sandström E. (1984). Susceptibility of *Neisseria gonorrhoeae* to rifampicin and thiamphenicol: correlation with protein I antigenic determinants. *Sex Trans Dis Suppl* **11:** 366–70.
20. Wølner-Hanssen P, Svensson L, Mårdh P-A, Weström L. (1985). Laparoscopic findings and contraceptive use in women with signs and symptoms suggestive of acute salpingitis. *Obstet Gynecol* **66:** 233–8.
21. Weström I. (1998). Decrease in incidence of women treated in hospital for acute salpingitis in Sweden. *Genitourin Med* **64:** 59–63.
22. Thorburn J. Ectopic pregnancy. The "epidemic" seems to be over. *Läkartidning 126:* **1:** 4701–6. (in Swedish with English summary).
23. Neuer A, Spandorfer SD, Giraldo P, Dieterle S, Rosenwaks Z, Witkin SS. (2000) The role of heat shock proteins in reproduction. *Hum Reprod Update*. **6:** 149–59.
24. Mårdh P-A, Johansson H, Svenningsen N. (1984). Intrauterine lung infection by *Chlamydia trachomatis* in a premature infant. *Acta Paed Scand* **73:** 569–572.
25. Svensson L-O, Mårdh P-A, Ahlgren M, Nordenskjöld F. (1985). Ectopic pregnancy and antibodies to *Chlamydia trachomatis*. *Fertil Steril* **414:** 313–7.
26. Mårdh P-A, Novikova D. Impact of chlamydial infections on pregnancy outcome, perinatal health and long-term sequelae of offsprings – a review of novel studies and reappraisal of earlier data. *J Obst Gyn.* In press.
27. Möller BR, Ahrons S, Laurin J, Mårdh P-A. (1982). Pelvic infection after elective abortion associated with *Chlamydia trachomatis*. *Obstet Gynecol* **59:** 210–13.
28. Osser S, Persson K. (1984). Postabortal pelvic infection associated with *Chlamydia trachomatis* and the influence of humoral immunity. *Am J Obstet Gynecol* **100:** 699–703.
29. Hallberg A, Mårdh P-A, Persson K, Ripa T. (1979). Pneumonia associated with *Chlamydia trachomatis* infection in an infant. *Acta Paed Scand* **68:** 765–7.
30. Mårdh P-A, Helin I, Bobeck S, Laurin J, Nilsson T. (1980). Colonisation of pregnant and puerperal women and neonates with *Chlamydia trachomatis*. *Br J Vener Dis* **56:** 96–100.
31. Brihmer C, Mårdh P-A, Osser S, Sikström B, Röbeck M, Wager U, Kallings I, Forselius A. (1996). Efficiency and safety of azithromycin versus lymecycline in genital chlamydial infection in non-pregnant women. *Scand J Infect Dis* **28:** 451–4.
32. Genc M, Mårdh P-A. (1996). A cost-effectiveness analysis of screening and treatment for *Chlamydia trachomatis* infection in asymptomatic women. *Ann Int Med* 124: 1–7.
33. Genc M, Ruusavaara L, Mårdh P-A. (1993). An economic evaluation of screening for *Chlamydia trachomatis* in adolescent males. *JAMA* **17:** 2057–64.

CHAPTER 10

Economic implications of
Chlamydia trachomatis

Mo Malek

Pharmacoeconomics Research Centre, University of St Andrews

Farzana Malik

Outcomes Research, Pfizer Pharmaceuticals, UK

INTRODUCTION

When referring to the economic implications of Chlamydia, we usually have two different types of economic issues in mind. The first is associated with the estimation of the overall impact on society of Chlamydia in terms of direct and indirect cost of disease. This is usually referred to as cost of illness or burden of illness and crucially depends on factors such as prevalence of the disease, the costs associated with the complications and how it affects the capacity of people to participate in productive work (see **Figure 1**).

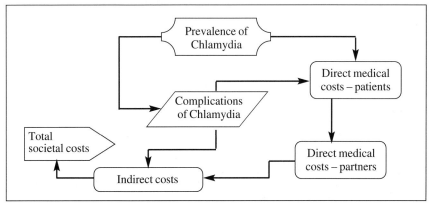

Figure 1. A cost of illness model for *Chlamydia trachomatis*.

Table 1: Economic Evaluation of Alternative Strategies of Managing Chlamydia
• Cost-effectiveness of:
screening strategies in women
screening in pregnant women
screening strategies in adolescent males
partner notification
empirical vs laboratory confirmed treatment
treatment regimens
• Cost-benefit evaluation of routine tests after treatment

The second category of economic issues arise from the economic evaluation of alternative strategies for the management of Chlamydia. The latter category covers a variety of issues some of which are presented in **Table 1**.

PREVALENCE AND INCIDENCE OF *CHLAMYDIA TRACHOMATIS*

Chlamydia trachomatis infection is the most common sexually transmitted bacterial disease in England and Wales[1]. The main features of this infection are threefold: infection is often asymptomatic, sequelae may be severe and if left untreated, infection can persist for more than a year[2]. Data from various surveys of individuals attending health services suggest infection may be asymptomatic in up to 70% of infected women[3,4] and in 4-11% of men[5,6]. The most serious sequelae of infection occurs in women where infection with *Chlamydia trachomatis* may lead to pelvic inflammatory disease (PID), ectopic pregnancy and infertility. These sequelae may have important lifetime consequences and are extremely costly to treat. According to the World Bank, chlamydial infection represents the most economically important sexually transmitted disease (STD) after HIV[6].

In the European region, approximately 10 million new cases of chlamydial infection occur each year[7]. Further, an estimated 600,000 cases per annum of salpingitis may be caused by *Chlamydia trachomatis* and approximately 120,000 cases will remain infertile. Prevalence rates collated for the European Region range between 1% and 33% in women who are screened and 10-20%

for men who undergo screening. Prevalence rates in persons with signs or symptoms of infection are much higher and may be as high as 80% in men with epidymitis and 70% in women with PID.

ECONOMIC BURDEN OF CHLAMYDIA

A landmark study of the economic burden of Chlamydia in the US population was conducted by Washington *et al* [8]. Interestingly, this study is still the only cost of illness study of Chlamydia published in the English language. Washington *et al* use the methodology of a prevalence-based approach to evaluate the cost of illness for Chlamydia. This type of methodology estimates the direct and indirect costs of Chlamydia accrued in a given year with the exception of future lost earnings of those patients who die as a result of Chlamydia (eg death from ectopic pregnancy). This study estimates healthcare costs for Chlamydia in men and for Chlamydia and its sequelae in women.

The economic burden was calculated as $1.4 billion dollars annually. When these costs are updated to 1998 values, they represent a total cost of $2.64 billion. The vast proportion of costs is attributed to the management of infections in women, and in particular the costs of managing the sequelae, mainly PID. Treatment of infections in women account for almost 80% of the total costs of treating Chlamydia.

Although this study demonstrates that Chlamydia represents a significant economic burden, the actual figures are likely to be an underestimate of the full costs of managing Chlamydia and its sequelae. The authors used the lower range of estimates for the direct healthcare costs of managing each of the Chlamydia and associated conditions. Secondly, the cost of managing complications in men (e.g. Reiter's syndrome) was excluded. Thirdly, infant costs exclude estimates for adverse pregnancy outcomes or mortality. Fourthly, costs of sequelae associated with asymptomatic infections were excluded even though up to 70% of infections in women and 30% in men are asymptomatic. Finally, the psychosocial costs of Chlamydia for patients, partners and the community were excluded.

Despite the exclusion of significant direct costs, Washington *et al* provide the best estimates of the economic burden of Chlamydia in the US. Similar studies have not been conducted in the UK or indeed in other English speaking countries. It is hoped that what follows will be found useful to those about to extend screening facilities and who propose to evaluate their cost-effectiveness.

COST-EFFECTIVENESS OF SCREENING STRATEGIES IN WOMEN

Asymptomatic infections represent 70% of *C. trachomatis* infections in women and 30% in men. It is vital therefore to identify and treat these infections before further transmission takes place. Various methods for the detection of asymptomatic infections are currently available. These methods include the use of different types of tests including culture tests and more recently, non-culture methods. Detection of asymptomatic chlamydial infection is a function of type of test, levels of sensitivity and specificity for the diagnostic test used, type of population and the expected prevalence rate in the population to be screened.

In a US study, Phillips *et al* [9] developed a model to evaluate the clinical and economic implications of testing for cervical infection caused by *C. trachomatis* infection in all women on routine gynaecological visits. The authors compared a strategy of routine testing using cell culture or rapid tests (DFA or EIA) with a strategy of no routine screening. It was suggested that the use of rapid tests followed by appropriate treatment in women with positive results would reduce overall costs where prevalence of *C. trachomatis* infection was 7% or more. When only direct costs are considered, the threshold value for rapid tests is a prevalence of 12%. The use of routine cultures would similarly reduce overall costs where prevalence of infection was 14% or greater. When only direct costs are considered, the threshold prevalence for culture is 25%. The authors conclude the choice of test should depend on the expected prevalence in the population, local costs and laboratory expertise.

Nettleman & Jones[10] evaluated the cost effectiveness of screening for women at moderate risk (7.9%) of urogenital infections with *C. trachomatis* in a US population. This study evaluated the economic impact of direct costs only from a societal perspective. The study conducted in two parts was unique in that it incorporated both clinical and economic evaluations. The first part was a clinical study of 434 sexually active college women to assess the sensitivity and specificity of three tests: microimmunoflurorescence, indirect fluorescent antibody assay and an enzyme-linked immunoassay. The second part of the study incorporated the development of a model to evaluate the cost-effectiveness of the three screening strategies compared to a strategy of no screening.

The results of the modelling exercise showed that screening all women with a direct antigen test costing less than $12 (1987 values) was more cost-effective than a strategy of no screening and no treatment. However, this was achieved with a high rate of false positive results, with only 53% of women with true positive results. Thus, treatment would be provided unnecessarily. Culture testing either alone or as a confirmatory procedure, was less cost-effective but had higher predictive values. Extensive sensitivity analysis revealed robustness of model for costs of tests, prevalence, complication rates for uncured infections and adverse events for antibiotic therapy.

In a study conducted in Sweden, Genc and Mardh[11] developed a model to evaluate the use of tissue cell culture, confirmed enzyme immunoassay, and DNA amplification assays by either polymerase chain reaction or ligase chain reaction. Treatment strategies used were doxycycline (7 day twice daily oral taken at home) and azithromycin (1g single dose, oral) administered under supervision. The authors used two decision trees to track outcomes of screening women and of tracing and treating sexual contacts of women with a positive diagnosis of *C. trachomatis*. Probability estimates were obtained from published literature. The study evaluated both direct medical costs and indirect societal costs. All costs related to delivery of healthcare and those attributed to lost wages and lost productivity were obtained from data published in Sweden.

The results of the modelling exercise showed that screening of women with any of the three diagnostic models was cost-effective, compared to no screening. DNA amplification combined with azithromycin treatment for patients with a positive test was the most cost-effective strategy, where prevalence of infection was at least 6%. Compared with no screening strategy, screening with enzyme immunoassay also generated savings and improved the cure rates but was less cost-effective than screening with DNA amplification. Compared with no screening, tissue culture was cost-effective only when the prevalence of infection is more than 14%. Treatment with doxycycline resulted in significantly lower cure rates than treatment with azithromycin due to patients' poor compliance with a twice-daily regimen for 7 days.

A more recent study[12] developed simple selective screening criteria for chlamydial infection in women to evaluate the contribution of clinical cervicitis to screening criteria and the cost-effectiveness of selective vs universal screening. The study included 31,025 women attending family practice and STD clinics in Washington, Oregon, Alaska and Idaho from 1989-1993. Different tests were evaluated according to where the women presented i.e. for women attending family clinics (11,141) a DFA test was used and for those women attending STD clinics (19,884), either a cell culture, DNA probe or EIA test was used for screening. The prevalence in this cohort of women was 6.6%. The study showed the independent predictors were: age

<20 yrs, signs of cervicitis, new sexual partner, multiple sexual partners and symptomatic partner. The risk factors were then used to develop selective screening criteria which were applied to a hypothetical cohort of one million Family Planning and STD patients. Finally, the authors conducted cost-effectiveness analysis to compare universal, selective screening with DFA and no screening in the hypothetical cohort of women. The authors calculated both direct and indirect societal costs. Indirect costs were those attributable to loss of productivity as a result of chlamydial infection. Intangible costs e.g. quality of life, pain, suffering were not included.

A sensitivity analysis was conducted to establish the threshold values above which universal screening would achieve savings compared to selective screening. Selective screening was cost-effective in both cohorts of women. However in family planning clinics, universal screening prevented more chlamydial cases than selective screening (47,025 vs 44, 674). This was at a higher cost and thus selective screening rather than universal screening was deemed to be the preferred option by the authors. In the STD setting, selective screening was also recommended. Sensitivity analysis showed the results of the analysis were robust with threshold values of 3.1%in family planning clinics and 6.9% in STD clinics. The use of a more expensive test e.g. LCR for screening had a minimal effect on the outcomes. The effect of using azithromycin, a more expensive but more effective therapy, was not evaluated by the authors.

In a Canadian study[13], the cost effectiveness of three different screening methods for early detection of *C. trachomatis* was evaluated. The model was constructed such that all women with a positive test were treated with either tetracycline or doxycycline, whose efficacy was assumed to be 95% and 100% respectively. Compliance rates for both regimens were assumed to be 70%. Literature was used to obtain complication rates for *C. trachomatis* infection which were similar to those used in other economic analyses. The study incorporated both direct medical and indirect societal costs. Direct costs were those incurred whilst testing, treating and managing costs of complications. Indirect costs were those associated with lost productivity of women as a result of chlamydial infection and its sequelae. This study showed that both DFA and enzyme immunoassay tests for early detection were cost-effective in women where prevalence was >6 or >7% respectively. Further, sensitivity analysis showed the probability of PID infection and cost of tests were the two variables which affected the outcome of the economic model.

COST-EFFECTIVENESS OF SCREENING IN PREGNANT WOMEN

Pregnant women are considered to be at high risk of *C. trachomatis* infection. The prevention of transmission to infants can result in the avoidance of additional costs incurred as a result of treating conjunctivitis and pneumonia in the babies. Additionally, prevention of transmission to the infant may result in lower mortality rates for newborns.

Nettleman and Bell[14] evaluated the cost-effectiveness of screening pregnant women for *C. trachomatis* by a third-party payer. Screening and treatment strategies are more complex in pregnant women as treatment options are more limited: Both mother and infant require therapy while sequelae for infection are more varied. The authors compared the direct medical costs associated with culture in all patients, followed by treatment for positive results, DFA in all patients followed by treatment for positive cases, or culture confirmation for positive DFA results and no screening tests. The treatment regimen was erythromycin for 7 days. Treatment for a single sexual partner was also included in the analysis. If the cost of DFA was less than US$6.30 (1990 values) or prevalence was >6.1% in pregnant women, routine screening with DFA followed by treatment for positive results was the most cost-effective option. Where the cost of DFA was <US$3.90 (1990 values) or the prevalence was higher than 6-7%, confirmation of positive DFA results followed by treatment was the more cost-effective strategy. And if the prevalence of infection was >14.8% or the cost of culture was less than US$7.50 (1990 values), culture followed by treatment for positive results was the preferred option. Where the mean cost of uncured infection was >US$284, DFA followed by treatment was the most cost-effective option. Sensitivity analysis showed that the variables affecting the outcome of results were prevalence of infection, cost of direct antigen test, cost of culture and mean cost of a persistent infection.

The authors of this study concluded that screening of pregnant women was not a cost-effective option in low prevalence populations (≤5%). The main disadvantage of this study was the use of charge data as a proxy for costs. However, it could be argued that from the perspective of the third-party payer, it is the charges incurred which represent the real burden of infection with *C. trachomatis,* according to the authors. Additionally, the authors did not allow for non-compliance of therapy with erythromycin in their estimation of efficacy of 92%.

COST-EFFECTIVENESS OF SCREENING STRATEGIES IN ADOLESCENT MALES

Adolescent males have the highest rates of infection and associated female complications compared with any other age groups[15-17]. Approximately 50% of nongonococcal urethritis infections and more than 50% of cases of epididymitis are caused by *C. trachomatis*[18]. Epididymitis is a serious condition which can occasionally lead to sterility. Further, this age group represents a major source of transmission to teenage girls.

Randolph & Washington[19] evaluated the costs and benefits of screening tests for Chlamydia in adolescent males. The authors developed a model to evaluate three screening methods in a hypothetical cohort of 1,000 sexually active adolescent males. The model considered direct medical costs only: treatment, screening, complications in sexual partners and complications in infected men. The results showed that the leukocyte esterase (LE) test had the lowest average cost-per-cure ($51) compared with direct-smear DFA ($192) and culture ($414). Compared with DFA, the authors estimated that the LE test would save more than $9,727 per cohort of 1,000 sexually active adolescent males, screened. The highest cure rates (56%) were achieved by the screening strategy, although they were more costly. DFA achieved cure rates of 51%, the LE test achieved cure rates of 49% and the no testing strategy achieved the lowest cure rates of 5%. A significant component of overall costs were those related to the treatment of infected female partners ($365 per infected case). Sensitivity analysis revealed robustness of model at clinically feasible values for major assumptions (prevalence, sensitivity, specificity of tests, PID rates, compliance, lost to follow-up rates). The analysis showed that the LE test would result in lower cost-per-cure and lower overall costs per cohort than culture and DFA at any prevalence of *C. trachomatis* infection. Compared to no screening, LE test would result in lower overall costs per cohort at prevalence rates >21%.

In an earlier study, Genc *et al*[20] evaluated the cost-effectiveness of identifying asymptomatic carriers of *C. trachomatis* in a hypothetical cohort of 1,000 adolescent males and their sexual partners/contacts. This study used a model to evaluate the impact of using enzyme immunoassay on either leukocyte esterase for positive urine samples (LE-EIA strategy) or on all urine samples (EIA strategy), compared with no screening strategy. Treatment regimens evaluated were doxycycline, 100 mg orally twice a day for seven days and azithromycin, 1g orally single dose. Analysis was carried out with the aid of two decision trees for all possible outcomes for both adolescent males and their sexual contacts. The study evaluated both direct and indirect medical costs. Direct costs were those related to costs of samples, tests, counselling sessions, appointments and treatment of initial *C. trachomatis* infection and its sequelae for both index cases and their partners. Indirect costs were those related to lost productivity as a result of participating in a healthcare programme.

The results showed, compared with no screening, that the LE-EIA and EIA screening strategies reduced the overall costs where the prevalence of Chlamydia was more than 2% and 10% respectively. The EIA strategy improved overall cure rates by 12% but reduced the incremental savings by at least $2,144 per cured male, compared with LE-EIA strategy. Confirmation of positive EIA tests reduced overall cost of the LE-EIA screening strategy where prevalence of *C. trachomatis* was less than 8%. In terms of antibiotic treatment, a single dose of azithromycin administered under supervision improved the cure rates of both screening strategies by 12-16% compared with a 7-day course of doxycycline, whilst reducing overall costs by 5-9%. However, the incremental cost-effectiveness ratios for the treatment strategies were not provided by the authors thus making an economic comparison difficult.

In summary, DFA screening was cost effective in populations >5% prevalence, and although cell culture has a higher predictive value, it is more costly. DNA amplification is more cost effective in populations with a prevalence of >6% than other models. The authors concluded that use of LE-EIA screening in combination with treatment of positive cases with azithromycin was the most cost-effective strategy, however in low risk populations, positive EIA tests should be confirmed.

COST-EFFECTIVENESS OF PARTNER NOTIFICATION

This is a situation where a third party e.g. healthcare personnel, take on the responsibility of informing the sexual partners of infected individuals and providing them with an evaluation of their exposure and treatment, if appropriate[21]. Katz *et al* [22] have published results of two studies which have evaluated the cost-effectiveness of using field follow-up for patients identified as having chlamydial infection as part of a screening process and female partners of men known to have had non-gonorrhoeal urethritis (NGU). The authors developed a decision analytic model to evaluate the cost-effectiveness of different options. However they did not state the perspective adopted for analysis. The inclusion of direct costs only, suggests the perspective of the STD clinic was adopted for the overall analysis. Costs for each strategy were determined from clinic personnel time, travel costs for healthcare personnel and other costs such as telephone calls made. A review of all the resources used for 40 culture-positive patients was made to determine resource use. Medical costs were taken from those reported in published literature.

The first study was carried out in an STD setting where patients were assigned to receive empirical antibiotic therapy for chlamydial infection or had urethral/endocervical specimens cultured. The latter group of patients was asked to return in a week's time to obtain the results; if positive they were asked to return for a follow-up appointment. For those patients who did not return after two weeks, a letter was sent out advising them of the status of their culture and asked to make an appointment. The results of these three groups of patients were then compared with the results obtained from using field follow-up in another group of patients. In this study, field follow-up consisted of an extensive interview of the infected patient by a disease intervention specialist followed by contact using a step-wise approach[23].

The results of the study showed that of 142 patients who had a positive *C. trachomatis* culture, approximately 34% (49) returned to obtain results and arrange a subsequent appointment. A total of 112 (79%) patients returned for treatment compared with 259/266 (97%) in the field follow-up group. The cost per patient of the field follow-up strategy was less than the reminder systems for both men and women.

In the second study, Katz *et al* compared the effectiveness of different methods for contacting females who were partners of men presenting with symptoms of NGU at an STD clinic. Over a six-month period, patients were randomised to receive counselling by a nurse for men to refer their sexual partners (n=217), or counselling by a disease specialist who obtained names of sexual contact but did not attempt to contact them (n=240) and field follow-up interview where the sexual partner was informed (n=221). The results from the second study revealed a significantly larger number of treated partners per index case (0.72) than nursing referral (0.22) and the interview strategy. The lowest costs per patient were achieved for the field follow-up group, followed by the nurse group and then the interview strategy group. Univariate sensitivity analysis revealed both models were robust for costs of each strategy and the cost of untreated chlamydial infection.

COST-EFFECTIVENESS OF TREATMENT: EMPIRICAL VS CONFIRMED LABORATORY DIAGNOSIS

Nettleman[10] compared the cost effectiveness of treating infected individuals who had a positive culture for *C. trachomatis* with those treated empirically i.e. based on signs and symptoms. The Diagnostic test used in this study was the cell culture method where specificity = 99% and sensitivity = 90% for men and 66-88% in women. Prevalence in the various sub-groups of patients were obtained from data on 22,063 patients who had attended an STD clinic in Indianapolis, USA between 1983-1984 and additionally from published literature. Patients were subgrouped according to high- or low-risk groups depending on their signs, symptoms and history. The appropriate antibiotic treatment used in the model, was at that time, deemed to be tetracycline 2g/day for 7 days (newer therapies were not yet available). This analysis was conducted from a third party payer and thus only direct medical costs were evaluated. The results showed empirical treatment was the most cost-effective option for all patients attending the STD clinic. However, if this option was not feasible, the next best alternative was empirical treatment of high-risk women and culture-based therapy for low-risk women. In men, the cost-effective option was that of empirical treatment in high-risk groups while in low-risk males performing no cultures and no therapy was the most cost-effective option.

COST-EFFECTIVENESS OF TREATMENT REGIMENS

A number of different antibiotic treatment regimens are available for the treatment of *C. trachomatis* as outlined in chapter 5. The availability of newer antibiotics such as the fluoroquinolones and azithromycin and cost containment measures by healthcare systems have led to research efforts to identify cost-effective treatment options. Newer drugs are more expensive than older, generic antibiotics, however they may offer the advantages of fewer side-effects and increased compliance with therapy when compared to traditional treatment options [24-26]. Nuovo *et al* [27] evaluated the cost-effectiveness of five different antibiotics for the treatment of *C. trachomatis* in non-pregnant women from the perspective of a healthcare system in California (erythromycin, tetracycline, doxycycline, ofloxacin, azithromycin). The authors developed a model and based their estimates of probability values and costs on published literature, state health plan reports and health insurance companies. Extensive sensitivity analysis was undertaken on the parameters: probability of PID and hospitalisation after treatment failure, cost of treatment for inpatient and outpatient PID, and cost and efficacy of azithromycin and doxycycline.

This model showed that the most cost-effective treatment regimes were the doxycycline and tetracycline strategies, followed by azithromycin, ofloxacin and erythromycin. In those patients who were non-compliant, azithromycin may be the best strategy because of the single dose, however, this was not accounted for in the analysis. Marra *et al*[28] criticised this study for its simplistic model. Further sequelae beyond PID (e.g. chronic pelvic pain, infertility and ectopic pregnancy) were not considered in the analysis. Additionally, the authors did not include the impact of non-compliance with older treatment regimens on the overall cure rates nor the costs incurred in managing adverse drug reactions. This is particularly pertinent as some of the older treatments such as erythromycin and tetracycline have been shown to have higher adverse events than newer agents[24,29]. Costs of treating secondary transmission to sexual partners were not considered in the analysis.

Haddix *et al*[30] also developed a model to evaluate the cost-effectiveness of treatment regimens for uncomplicated chlamydial infection. The authors compared treatment with azithromycin 1g with doxycycline 100 mg twice daily for 7 days in a cohort of 10,000 non-pregnant women. Additionally, the authors evaluated the treatments based on two diagnostic strategies; laboratory-confirmed *C. trachomatis* infection and presumptive diagnosis, based on clinical signs and symptoms.

This study evaluated the economic impact from the perspectives of the US healthcare system and the publicly funded clinic. In the latter perspective, costs related to sequelae of infection would be managed on an out-patient basis. Probability estimates were obtained from published clinical trials. The effectiveness of doxycycline was adjusted for a compliance rate of 80%, and non-compliant patients were assumed to be treatment failures. For azithromycin, compliance was assumed to be 100% since it is a single dose regimen and was administered in the clinics. The costs included in the model were those relating to treatment, treatment of PID and its sequelae (chronic pelvic pain, ectopic pregnancy and infertility). Costs for sequelae which would occur in future years were discounted at an annual rate of 5%. Costs relating to PID were taken from Washington and Katz (1991)[31]. Additionally, the model assumed 25% of women with tubal-factor infertility would seek treatment. Sensitivity analysis was carried out for prevalence rate of infection in those women treated presumptively, doxycycline compliance rates, cost of PID and its sequelae, probabilities of developing PID in compliant and non-compliant patients, and the risk of developing further sequelae.

The results from the healthcare payer perspective revealed that the use of azithromycin would cost an additional US$290k (1993 values) to treat chlamydial infections in a cohort of 10,000 women under a laboratory confirmed strategy, resulting in savings of US$1.2 million for treating the PID that had been prevented. In the presumptively treated model, use of azithromycin would cost an additional US$290k and would save US$240k to treat a cohort of 10k women. This would result in incremental cost savings of US$800 per additional case of PID prevented for azithromycin versus doxycycline in treated patients. Extensive sensitivity analysis revealed the robustness of model to the extent that azithromycin achieved savings for all plausible values. However, the results of the presumptive model were more sensitive to changes in probability and cost estimates used in the model.

From the perspective of the public health clinic, azithromycin would cost an additional US$220k (1993 values) for a cohort of 10k women in a laboratory-confirmed model, but would result in savings of US$29k from reduced treatment costs of PID. This would result in net savings of US$709 per additional case of PID prevented. In the presumptive treatment model, azithromycin treatment would cost an additional US$220k but would save US$5,670 from reduced treatment costs of PID. This would result in net costs of US$3,969 per additional case of PID prevented. Sensitivity analysis for both strategies revealed that azithromycin becomes more cost-effective in public clinics with non-compliant populations and where prevalence of *C. trachomatis* infection is higher. The authors concluded that the use of azithromycin is more cost-effective under laboratory confirmed conditions from the healthcare-system perspective. In patients who are presumptively treated, azithromycin continues to be cost-effective resulting in incremental cost savings of US$800 (1993 values) per case of PID prevented. Although, azithromycin is cost-effective, from the perspective of a publicly funded clinic, only a small percentage of treatment costs relating to PID and its sequelae is incurred by the clinic; thus this option is also more expensive. The remainder of the costs incurred in treatment of PID and its sequelae will be absorbed by other public or non-public organisations; thus from a societal perspective, such savings are non-existent or artificial.

Marra *et al*[28] further developed the models constructed by Haddix *et al*[30] to evaluate the cost-effectiveness of azithromycin and doxycycline from the perspective of the Canadian healthcare system for a cohort of 5,000 non-pregnant women. The costs of managing complications of PID are lower in the Canadian system (the justification used by Marra for developing this model). Probability estimates and costs for resources were obtained from the literature, hospital costing departments and expert opinion. The results showed that azithromycin in a laboratory confirmed model would result in savings of Can$279,150 (1995 values) for a cohort of 5,000 women. In the presumptively treated model, use of azithromycin would result in savings of Can$1,700 for this cohort. In conclusion, the authors state that widespread use of azithromycin in Canada for laboratory confirmed cases of *C. trachomatis* would result in savings of Can$3 million in direct medical expenses per year. However there are a number of limitations to studies conducted by both Haddix *et al* and Marra *et al*; the cost of managing adverse effects of antibiotic therapy were not included; cost of secondary transmission to sexual partners was not evaluated; different screening strategies were not evaluated; and both models evaluate direct medical costs only. Thus the full economic impact from a societal perspective has not been evaluated.

Finally, Magid *et al*[32] conducted an economic evaluation very similar to that of Haddix *et al* and Marra *et al* in evaluating the impact of azithromycin compared to doxycycline in the treatment of women with *C. trachomatis* infection. The advantage of this study over the two previous studies is that it includes the impact of adverse events related to treatment with antibiotics and the costing of sequelae which occur as a result of secondary transmission of infection. Additionally, Magid *et al* identified cure rates for different levels of non-compliance with doxycycline. The results of this study were similar to Haddix *et al* and Marra *et al*. When base-case assumptions are used, azithromycin was the more cost-effective treatment option for uncomplicated *C. trachomatis* infection in women. Azithromycin resulted in a reduction in major complications of infection by 2,392 compared to doxycycline at approximately 57% of the cost per patient. Nevertheless, the authors recognised that the higher initial cost of acquiring azithromycin may limit widespread use of this treatment option in the essentially fragmented healthcare system in North America.

COST-BENEFIT EVALUATION OF A TEST-OF-CURE - STRATEGY

The value of routine tests after treatment of infection is unclear. Guidelines in the majority of countries do not recommend a test of cure although the majority of GUM physicians in Great Britain offer the service to patients[33]. A Norwegian study used a model to evaluate the cost-benefit of a test-of-cure strategy in a hypothetical cohort of 10,000 women with a positive diagnosis of *C. trachomatis* infection[34]. The tests used were either cell culture of a rapid test or a no-test-of-cure strategy for those who failed initial therapy. In this model, patients were continually cycled until all patients were cured under the test-of-cure strategy. This study evaluated direct costs only, diagnostic tests, repeat physician visits, antibiotic therapy and treatment of sequelae. The analysis was conducted from a third party payer perspective. The antibiotic used was lymecycline 100mg orally twice a day, a cheaper alternative to doxycyline at an assumed effectiveness of 95%. The results of the analysis demonstrated that the costs of a test-of-cure strategy were approximately twice that of a no-test-of-cure strategy. Sensitivity analysis revealed the model was robust to changes in the sensitivity and specificity of tests used with assumed specificity of 98% and sensitivity of 80%, however this was dependent on estimates of the efficacy of lymecycline. Non-compliance with therapy was not factored into the analysis. Additionally, costs of treating sexual partners, infants, male infertility and indirect costs associated with lost productivity as a result of test-of-cure were not incorporated in the analysis. Although this study is titled 'cost-benefit-analysis', it does not attempt to value the benefits of testing the patients. Like the CDC, the authors recommended that a test of cure is not required. In those cases where a test of cure is required either for research or other purposes, Black[35] has recommended the use of cell culture methods due to their positive predictive value in a treated population where prevalence is likely to be low.

SUMMARY AND CONCLUSION

Chlamydial infections represent a significant economic burden. Asymptomatic infections account for between 30% and 70% of infections. Detection and appropriate management of asymptomatic infections may lead to a reduction in the total costs of treating Chlamydia and its sequelae. Women account for a significant component of the total costs of Chlamydia, especially the costs of complications such as PID. Additionally, adolescent males represent a high-risk population and a major source of transmission to young women. A variety of diagnostic tests are available for detection of asymptomatic infections. Economic evaluations suggest screening of asymptomatic individuals is a cost-effective strategy, particularly in adolescent males and in young women. Further, treatment of chlamydial infections with a single dose of azithromycin appears to be the most cost-effective treatment strategy. The extent of a reduction in societal costs is a function of the types of tests used and the expected prevalence in the population being screened.

REFERENCES

1. Communicable Disease Report (1998). 'Sexually transmitted diseases quarterly report: genital infection with *Chlamydia trachomatis* in England and Wales' **6**(22).
2. Brunham RC. (1990), 'A General Model of Sexually Transmitted Disease Epidemiology and its Implications for Control' in *Medical Clinics in North America* **74**(6):1339–52.
3. Zimmerman H, Potterat J, Dukes R, Muth J *et al.* (1990). 'Epidemiological differences between Chlamydia and Gonorrhea' *Am J Public Health* **80**:1338–42.
4. Lycke E *et al.* (1980). 'The risk of transmission of genital *Chlamydia trachomatis* infection is less than that of genital Neisseria gonorrhoeae infection' in *Sex Trans Dis* **7**(1): 6–10.
5. Karam G, Martin D, Flote T *et al.* (1995). 'Asymptomatic *Chlamydia trachomatis* infections among sexually active men' *J Infect Dis* **154**: 900–03.
6. World Bank (1993) World Development Report 1993. Investing in health. Oxford: Oxford University Press, 1993.
7. Mardh PA and Westrom LA. Working Group Report on Chlamydial Infections. Sweden (unpublished document) Ref EUR/ICP/CDS 199 (243 8G)
8. Washington A *et al.* (1987). '*Chlamydia trachomatis* Infections in the United States: what are they costing us?' in *JAMA* **257**: 2070–72.
9. Phillips R *et al.* (1990). 'Should tests for *Chlamydia trachomatis* cervical infection be done during routine Gynecologic visits?' in *Annals of Internal Medicine* **107**: 188–194.
10. Nettleman M and Jones R. (1988). 'Cost-effectiveness of screening women at moderate risk for genital infections caused by *Chlamydia trachomatis*' in *JAMA* **260**(2): 207–213.
11. Genc M and Mardh P. (1996). 'A Cost-effectiveness Analysis of Screening and Treatment for *Chlamydia trachomatis* Infection in Asymptomatic Women' in *Ann Intern Med* **124**(1):1–7.
12. Marrazzo J *et al.* (1999). 'Performance and cost-effectiveness of selective screening criteria for *Chlamydia trachomatis* infection in women' in *Sex Trans Dis* **24**(3): 131–141.
13. Estany A. *et al.* (1989). 'Early detection of genital chlamydial infection in women: an economic evaluation' in *Sex Trans Dis* **16**(1):21–27.
14. Nettleman M and Bell T. (1991). 'Cost-effectiveness of prenatal testing for *Chlamydia trachomatis*' in *Am J Obstet Gynecol* **164**(5): 1289–94.
15. Washington A, Sweet R and Shafer M-A. (1985). 'Pelvic inflammatory disease and its sequelae in adolescents' in *J Adolescent health Care* **6**: 298–310.
16. Stamm W *et al.* (1984). '*Chlamydia trachomatis* urethral infections in men' in *Annals of Internal Medicine* **100**: 47–51.
17. Handsfield H, Jasman L,. Roberts P *et al.* (1986). 'Criteria for selective screening for *Chlamydia trachomatis* infection in women attending family planning clinics' *JAMA* **255**: 1730–34.
18. Thomson S and Washington A. ' Epidemiology of sexually transmitted *Chalmydia trachomatis* infections in Epidemiology Review, **5**: 96–123.
19. Randolph A and Washington E. (1990). 'Screening for *Chlamydia trachomatis* in adolescent males: a cost-based decision analysis' in *AJPH* **80**(5): 545–550.

20. Genc M, Ruusuvaara L and Mardh P. (1993). 'An economic evaluation of screening for *Chlamydia trachomatis* in adolescent males' in *JAMA* **270**(17): 2057–64.
21. MMWR (1993). 'Recommendations for the Prevention and Management of *Chlamydia trachomatis* Infections, 1993' *MMWR*, **42**(12): 1–39.
22. Katz B *et al.* (1988). 'Efficiency and cost-effectiveness of field follow-up for patients with *Chlamydia trachomatis* infection in a sexually transmitted diseases clinic' in *Sex Trans Dis* **15**:11–16.
23. Marra C *et al.* (1998). '*Chlamydia trachomatis* in Adolescents and Adults: clinical and economic implications' in *Pharmacoeconomics* **13**(2): 191–222.
24. Hopkins S. (1991). 'Clinical toleration and safety of azithromycin' in *Am J Med* **91** Suppl. 3A: 40–5.
25. Bauchmann LH, Stephens J, Richey CM, *et al.* (1996). 'Measured versus self-reported compliance with doxycyline therapy for *Chlamydia* associated syndromes (abstract) 36th Interscience Conference on Antimicrobial agents and Chemotherapy, Sep 15-18; New Orleans: 256.
26. Augenbraun M, *et al.* (1996). 'Compliance with Doxycyline Therapy in an STD clinic' (abstract) 36th Interscience Conference on Antimicrobial agents and Chemotherapy, Sep 15-18; New orleans: Abstract No 37.
27. Nuovo J *et al.* (1995). 'Cost effectiveness analysis of five different antibiotic regimens for the treatment of uncomplicated *Chlamydia trachomatis* cervitis' in *J Am Board Fam Pract* **8**(1): 7–16.
28. Marra F, Marra C and Patrick D. (1997.) 'Cost effectiveness of azithromycin and doxycyline for *Chlamydia trachomatis* infection in women: a Canadian perspective' in *Can J Infec Dis* **8**(4): 202–208.
29. Bowie W *et al.* (1982). 'Efficacy of treatment regimens for lower urogenital *Chlamydia trachomatis* infection in women' in *Am J Obstet Gynecol* **142**(2): 125–129.
30. Haddix A, Hillis S and Kassler W. (1995). 'The cost-effectiveness of azithromycin for *Chlamydia trachomatis* infections in women' in *Sex Trans Dis* **22**(5): 274–280.
31. Washington AE, Katz P. (1991). Cost of and payment source for pelvic inflammatory disease. Trends and projections, 1983 through 2000. *JAMA* **266**(18): 2565–9.
32. Magid D, Douglas J and Schwartz S. (1996). 'Doxycyline Compared with Azithromycin for Treating Women with Genital *Chlamydia trachomatis* Infections: an Incremental Cost-effectiveness Analysis' in *Ann Intern Med* **124**: 389–399.
33. Radcliffe KW, Rowen D, Mercey DE et. al. (1990) 'Is a test of cure necessary following tratment for cervical infection with *Chlamydia trachomatis* ?' *Genitourin Med* **66**: 444–46.
34. Schiotz H and Csango P. (1992). 'Test-of-Cure for asymptomatic genital infections in women: a cost-benefit analysis' in *Sex Trans Dis* May-June:133–136.
35. Black C. (1997). 'Current methods of laboratory diagnosis of *Chlamydia trachomatis* infections' in *Clin Microbiol* reviews, Jan:pp160–184.

CHAPTER 11

Is the global elimination of
trachoma feasible?

Sohrab Darougar
University of London, UK

Timothy R Moss
Genito-Urinary Medicine, Doncaster Royal Infirmary

Dayshad Darougar
Research Assistant

INTRODUCTION

In 1998, the World Health Organization (WHO) adopted a resolution for the Global Elimination of Trachoma (GET) by the year 2020[1]. Subsequently the WHO Alliance for the global elimination of trachoma (GET Alliance) has taken the initiative for coordinating trachoma control programmes of member countries, to mobilise resources required and to develop technologies, strategies and policies for achieving the aim of GET by the year 2020[1]. The GET Alliance consist of representatives of governments, non-government agencies, charities, academics, research organisations, pharmaceutical companies and other institutions with interest in community healthcare and WHO representatives.

The knowledge, experience and expertise gained by the WHO during the eradication of smallpox, the elimination of poliomyelitis as a major public health problem and in controlling major preventable infections is the subject of international respect. This expertise in combination with modern technologies and more effective anti-trachoma drugs has led to confidence that the goal of eliminating trachoma by the year 2020 is achievable. However, a number of clinicians, scientists and health specialists believe that the objective of GET by the year 2020 may possibly be compromised, because of the absence of adequate financial and human resources and lack of political commitment in some of the developing countries where trachoma is hyperendemic.

In this chapter we examine important features of trachoma complex. We also discuss a range of therapeutic interventions and their potential impact on the success or failure of GET programme.

Trachoma is one of the oldest and most common eye diseases worldwide. The disease and its blinding complications were known in China in the 27th century BC, in Sumaria in the 21st Century BC, in Greece in the 5th century BC and Rome in the 1st century BC. Trachoma was extremely common in Greece and the Middle-East during the medieval period. In Europe, trachoma was spread by crusaders returning from Palestine and after the Napoleonic wars. However, trachoma in Europe and Northern America disappeared in the early 20th century. It is interesting to note that trachoma was eradicated from Europe and Northern America long before active anti-trachoma drugs became available.

CAUSE

Trachoma is caused by *Chlamydia trachomatis* (CT) an obligate intra-cellular bacteria. The CT serotypes causing trachoma are A, B, Ba and C. However occasionally CT serotypes D and E (common genital pathogens) have been isolated from the eyes with trachoma. the original *Chlamydia pneumoniae* isolates; TW-183 and IOL-207 were isolated from the eyes of children with trachoma in Taiwan and Iran respectively[2]. The role of *C. pneumoniae* in causing trachoma has not been established. Serological studies in Iran showed that the child and some members of his family had type-specific IgG to IOL-207, whereas other children in the adjacent families had no antibodies to IOL-207. The potential pathogenicity of the IOL-207 isolate in causing eye disease was shown in a laboratory accident[3]. A technologist who was propagating IOL-207 isolate in eggs and cell cultures was accidentally infected with the agent and developed a severe keratoconjunctivitis. The eye infection was cured after intensive topical and systemic treatment with tetracyclines exceeding one month. In this patient, cell culture failed to detect the causative organism. Eventually IOL-207 was isolated after inoculation of conjunctival specimens into hens' fertile eggs and passing several times. Concurrently, IOL-207 was also isolated from the yolk-sac of fertile eggs after inoculating with infected cell culture materials and repeated passing of egg cultures.

Serological tests on this patient showed absence of Chlamydia antibodies in blood collected before the infection and presence of type-specific IgG to IOL-207 and four-fold rising titre of IgG after the infection.

CLINICAL FEATURES

Trachoma is a chronic infection of the conjunctiva and cornea (keratoconjunctivitis). Pathological changes may also develop in the sub-epithelial connective tissues, tarsal plates, lacrymal gland and ducts, nasal mucosa, pre-auricular lymph nodes and in the upper respiratory tract. The disease generally affects both eyes.

Incubation period
The incubation period of trachoma remains unclear. In experimental inoculation of the eye of human volunteers with trachoma agents, the incubation period was between 1 to 3 weeks. In rural communities, CT was isolated from the eyes of 6 week old babies[4]. This may suggest that under those conditions the incubation period may be less than six weeks[4].

Symptoms
Common symptoms of trachoma may include watering, mucopurulent discharge, redness, irritation, discomfort, itching and foreign body sensation. In advanced cases of trachoma and particularly in those with severe scarring, patients may complain of heavy and thick lids, dryness, moderate to severe foreign body sensation and blurred vision. In rural communities with high prevalence of trachoma and bacterial conjunctivitis, patients generally do not consider the above symptoms as abnormal, and hence do not complain.

Signs
Clinical signs may occur in the palpebral and bulbar conjunctiva, limbus and cornea.

In the palpebral conjunctiva the major signs are hyperaemia, diffuse infiltration, papillae, follicles and scarring. Papillae may present in various forms. At early stages, they appear as small red spots in the conjunctiva. At later stages, they are much larger, each containing a dense collection of inflammatory cells around congested vessels in a thickened conjunctiva.

Follicles may vary in size and presentation. In the early stages of infection, the follicles are generally small and may appear as yellowish to grey-white nodules against a background of red papillae. However in chronic trachoma, the follicles (particularly in the fornices) may become very large. The follicles contain a collection of inflammatory cells. In well developed follicles, the inflammatory cells are organised around a germinal centre.

Conjunctival scars may develop with variable intensity and shape. In mild cases, scars may appear as fine, focal or linear, while in severe cases they may present as diffuse or synechial or as a broad fibrovascular membrane.

Limbal signs may include vascular congestion, diffuse infiltration, transient follicles and depressions called Herbert's pits.

Corneal signs may include focal or circumcorneal vascularisation, punctate epithelial keratitis, sub-epithelial punctate keratitis, diffuse infiltration and corneal scar. Pannus, the specific corneal sign of trachoma consist of corneal vascularisation with punctate epithelial and punctate sub-epithelial keratitis and diffuse infiltration between vessels. At early stages of trachoma, pannus is small and may be detected only by slit-lamp or high magnification lens. In advanced cases of trachoma, pannus is generally visible to the naked eye.

Complications

Trachoma complications may be categorised as blinding and non-blinding. Blinding complications may include severe conjunctival scarring, severe sub-conjunctival and peri-tarsal fibrosis and tarsal degeneration which may cause lid deformity, trichiasis and entropion. The entropion and trichiasis cause misdirected lashes to abrade the cornea, leading to infected corneal ulcers, scarring and ultimately loss of vision. Non-blinding complications may include dry eye, corneal and conjunctival keratinisation, post-trachomatous cystic degeneration and symblepharon (conjunctival synechiae). The blinding complications generally occur in the older age group and mostly affect the population over the age of sixty.

Clinical variants

In hyperendemic areas, trachoma may present in various clinical forms. The classical form of trachoma consists of the presence of various amounts of papillae and follicles in the palpebral conjunctiva and active pannus. It is common in pre-school children. In young babies under one year, trachoma may present as moderate to severe papillary conjunctivitis resembling bacterial conjunctivitis. Follicles generally appear in older babies and become prominent in pre-school children. In older school children, scarring may appear in addition to follicles, papillae, diffuse infiltration in the conjunctiva and pannus. In adolescents and adults, scarring may be the main feature of trachoma. However, in adults (mainly female) who are living in large families with several young children with active trachoma, follicles and papillae may be found along with the conjunctival scarring.

In communities with a low prevalence of trachoma, clinical forms are different from those in hyperendemic areas. Mild and moderate papillary trachoma are common in older babies and in pre-school children. Mild follicular trachoma is mainly found in children aged between 4 and 10 years. Mild focal scarring may develop in school children and adults. In these communities the disease is classified as non-blinding trachoma, because of the absence or very low prevalence of severe scarring, entropion and trichiasis.

Natural history

Trachoma is generally considered as a chronic keratoconjunctivitis which may last for several years. It is stated that trachoma may start as a mild or moderate papillary conjunctivitis with a few small follicles progressing towards a florid trachoma with large papillae, mature follicles and pannus. At a later stage, fine, focal or linear scars may develop alongside papillae and follicles in the palpebral conjunctiva. In a late or inactive trachoma, follicles and papillae are no longer present but scars and/or fibrovascular membrane are present in part or whole of the palpebral conjunctiva. However, with better understanding of immunopathological processes, substantial changes in the natural history of trachoma have been identified, particularly in relation to its reduced pressure of transmission. This modified natural history of trachoma has been observed in most communities.

Experimental inoculations of the eye of human volunteers with trachoma agent have shown that infection starts as a moderate papillary conjunctivitis, progressing into a follicular conjunctivitis. The ocular infection generally lasts up to three months and is followed by spontaneous recovery without treatment. It is interesting that none of these volunteers developed pannus or scars.

Experimental studies in laboratory animals inoculated with their own natural chlamydial pathogens or in non-human primates inoculated with CT have shown that:

- primary infection recovered spontaneously in the course of a few weeks without treatment. Non of the inoculated animals developed conjunctival scarring or pannus.
- When the animals were inoculated repeatedly, the eyes developed a

chronic conjunctivitis lasting for several months or longer. Conjunctival scarring and corneal vascularisation developed in most of the eyes.

In communities with low prevalence of active trachoma, where pressure of transmission and rate of re-infection are low, the natural history of trachoma is different from those communities with hyperendemic trachoma and high prevalence of severe trachoma. The differences in low prevalence areas include:

- primary trachoma occurs in older babies and in young children
- in pre-school and school children, trachoma presents as a mild follicular conjunctivitis and its prevalence is low
- in most of the older school children and adolescents, trachoma recovers spontaneously without causing scarring or pannus or may produce mild scarring
- the prevalence of newly developed blinding complications of trachoma including trichiasis, entropion and corneal scarring are very low.

In conclusion, trachoma in communities with low prevalence of active trachoma is no longer considered as a blinding disease.

EPIDEMIOLOGY

Trachoma is the most prevalent eye disease worldwide and is second to cataract in causing blindness. Trachoma is considered a major health problem in the rural communities of dry and hot regions of North, East and South Africa, the Middle East, Northern India and South-East Asia. Foci of endemic trachoma also exist in some areas of South America, Australia and some of the tropical and sub-tropical Pacific islands.

Incidence
It is difficult to quantify the incidence of trachoma in the rural communities. This is due to the exacerbation of signs in patients with mild trachoma following re-infection, the masking of clinical signs during seasonal outbreaks of bacterial conjunctivitis or relapse of trachoma in patients who have been treated. However, studies in communities with high prevalence of active trachoma have shown:

- The incidence of trachoma in babies is very high. In babies under the age of one, approximately 50% develop trachoma and by the age of two, over 80% may have trachoma.

- The incidence of trachoma in villages untouched by trachoma control programmes may be as high as 20% per annum.
- The incidence of new cases of trachoma in the rural communities who have been treated with topical or systemic drugs was between 5 to 15% per annum.

In communities with low prevalence of active trachoma, the incidence of trachoma is very low, because of the low level of shedding of trachoma agent from a smaller reservoir of infection. This results in a low rate of transmission in the community.

Prevalence

A few decades ago, the WHO estimated that about 500 million people were suffering from trachoma. Recently the WHO revised the global prevalence of trachoma and estimated that approximately 150 million people have active trachoma, over 10 million are suffering from entropion/trichiasis, six million are blind in both eyes and that over 10 million are blind in one eye or have low vision due to trachoma.

The prevalence of trachoma varies considerably. In most countries of the Middle-East, Indian sub-continent, South-East Asia, Latin America and Australia, the prevalence of active trachoma has decreased substantially due to economic, environmental and public health improvements. In these countries, the overall prevalence of active trachoma is at present estimated to be less than 30%, with the rate of severe trachoma in children less than 10%.

In rural areas of North, East and South Africa where trachoma is still hyperendemic, up to 50% of the population may have active trachoma. Of these, 10 to 20% are suffering from severe trachoma. In pre-school children in these areas, the prevalence of active trachoma may be as high as 70%, with the prevalence of entropion/trichiasis as high as 10%. In adults over the age of 60, entropion/trichiasis may reach 50%[5].

Age

In areas where trachoma is hyperendemic, active trachoma can be detected in 2 to 3 month old babies. In pre-school children, trachoma may be present in up to 70% and over 50% of them may have moderate to severe trachoma. In older children and those attending schools, the prevalence of trachoma declines gradually and active trachoma may be present only in a minority of children. In adults, active trachoma is commonly associated with conjunctival scarring and may be present in 5 to 40%. Laboratory studies have shown that a large number of pre-school children are shedding detectable trachoma agent and as such they are a major reservoir of infection[5].

In communities with a low prevalence of trachoma, babies are commonly free of trachoma. In pre-school children, the disease is mild. In older children, only a minority have a mild trachoma and most adults show no signs of active trachoma or severe conjunctival scarring.

Sex

In pre-school children the prevalence and severity of trachoma is similar in both sexes. In older children and young adults, females have a markedly higher prevalence of active trachoma and more severe disease than males. In older women, the prevalence of trachoma and its blinding complications (ie entropion and trichiasis) are at least 2 to 3 times higher than in older men[6].

Family and village distribution

Both the prevalence and severity of trachoma are generally higher in large families with three or more young children. In these families, almost all children may have active trachoma. Most suffer from moderate to severe disease. Young mothers of these children, commonly have active trachoma with moderate to severe scarring. Older members of these families (and in particular females) may have more entropion, trichiasis, corneal opacity or blindness compared with those in families with two or less young children. Prevalence and severity of trachoma is lower in villages with a small population, in villages with scattered houses and in those with accessible clean water. Trachoma is uncommon among nomads who have small and widely scattered family units[4].

In villages, trachoma is generally distributed in clusters. The prevalence and severity of trachoma is higher among groups of families living in large houses or in houses built close to each other. Distribution of trachoma in clusters within the village has been shown by serotyping of CT or by detecting type-specific IgG to CT agent. In a study in Southern Iran, it was found that a particular CT serotype was present in a cluster of families in one part of the village and that a majority of members of the families within the cluster showed type-specific IgG to the same serotype. A second cluster of families living in another part of the village were infected with a different CT serotype and members of these families had type-specific IgG to that serotype (Treharne *et al* unpublished data).

Reservoir of CT
Babies and pre-school children constitute a large reservoir of infection[4,6]. In areas with high prevalence of trachoma, over 50% of babies and most pre-school children have moderate to severe trachoma. In these cases, CT has been isolated commonly from their conjunctival specimens, occasionally from ocular and nasal discharges and infrequently from the throat. Older children and young adults with active trachoma and women with severe chronic disease may occasionally shed CT and as such may remain a reservoir of infection. However, eyes of infants and young children are the major reservoirs of CT.

Transmission
There is no intermediate host for transmission of trachoma. In rural communities, infectious eye and nose discharges containing CT may be transmitted by hands, face to face contacts, by cloths used to remove eye and nasal discharges, bedding where children are sleeping in one bed and by house flies.

Studies have shown that eye seeking house flies, *Musca domestica* and to a greater degree *Musca sorbens* can transmit infectious materials from eye to eye. In a study in Southern Iran, flies have successfully transmitted a colour marker from eyes of children to the face and eyes of other children playing nearby within 30 minutes[4]. In a laboratory study, CT was isolated from the legs and proboscis of flies fed on CT infected materials. In the villages, control of houseflies led to a substantial decrease in the prevalence and incidence of trachoma[7].

It is suggested that children who have had severe trachoma and who are exposed to repeated re-infection and adults with severe scarring, trichiasis and entropion who are economically under-privileged are at risk of remaining locked in a vicious circle of repeated transmission of infection from children to children, children to adults and adults to children. This is a particular problem for those living in large families with several young children, where an unhygienic environment also facilitates transmission[4].

CONTROL OF TRACHOMA

In the past few decades, a number of countries in Africa, the Middle-East and South East Asia have established with WHO support, national programmes for control of trachoma. It is reported that in some of these countries, trachoma control programmes have been successful in reducing the prevalence of trachoma and its blinding complications. A number of experts and clinicians have challenged these claims. They argue that most of these programmes relied almost entirely on the efficacy of intermittent application of tetracycline eye ointment for interrupting transmission of trachoma and less on sanitation, health education and establishing a basic primary healthcare network. It is also suggested that mass therapy with topical antibiotic was not entirely successful, because of the erratic and inadequate supply of tetracycline eye ointment at the point of use, inability of individuals to apply eye ointment correctly to their own eyes or in the eyes of their children, and lack of compliance by villagers. They also point out that where reduction of trachoma has been achieved, this was mostly due to improvements in the economy of the country as a whole (for example: oil producing countries), better standards of housing, sanitation, schooling and the development of a primary healthcare system in the rural areas.

To control trachoma *with the aim of its elimination*, there is a need for protecting susceptible persons, stopping shedding of the agent by infected cases, interrupting the transmission of CT between persons or by involving all of these measures together.

There is no natural immunity to trachoma. Acquired immunity may develop which provides a partial or transient protection. Patients with active trachoma are susceptible to re-infection. In these patients, re-exposure to CT may produce a more severe follicular response and pannus and enhance development of conjunctival and sub-conjunctival diffuse cellular infiltration, scarring and sub-epithelial fibrosis. In patients with healed trachoma, re-exposure to live CT or its antigenic components may enhance development of lid deformity, trichiasis and entropion.

At present there is no effective anti-trachoma vaccine available. Early attempts to develop a trachoma vaccine and subsequently to immunise populations in Taiwan, Iran and Egypt showed only a mild and transient protection against trachoma. In addition, it was found that vaccinated groups developed delayed hypersensitivity and when further exposed to CT, they developed more severe trachoma in comparison to those who had not been vaccinated[8].

Interruption of transmission can be achieved by health education, provision of accessible clean water, improved housing, hygiene, public healthcare and waste disposal. These improvements can substantially and permanently reduce the prevalence and incidence of trachoma, but require substantial financial resources and may take several years to produce a tangible effect.

Mass therapy of communities with hyperendemic trachoma or treatment of individuals in communities with a low prevalence of active trachoma using effective anti-chlamydial antibiotics may stop shedding of CT. In order to achieve a substantial and lasting reduction in CT shedding in the community, it is essential to find a drug and/or a delivery system which requires a single application only with a minimum of supervision. This must be affordable by poor countries. It must also be possible to provide re-treatment annually for several years.

GLOBAL ELIMINATION OF TRACHOMA

Since 1996, the WHO GET Alliance has convened several meetings to develop policies, strategies, procedures and technologies required for the global elimination of trachoma by the year 2020. During these meetings, it was proposed and agreed that a number of member countries with WHO support, should implement the following operational research projects in order to develop highly effective and practical programmes for elimination of trachoma:

Operational Research Projects
Rapid trachoma assessment
The following simple method for rapid assessment and recording of the presence and severity of trachoma, trichiasis and entropion has been recommended for field evaluation:[9]

TF Presence of follicles in the upper tarsal conjunctiva.
TI (intensive or severe trachoma) – This is diagnosed by the presence of papillae and diffuse infiltration masking more than half of the palpebral conjunctival vessels.
TS Trachoma with scarred conjunctiva
TT Presence of entropion and trichiasis
CO Corneal opacity

The practicality and validity of this rapid assessment method was tested under the field conditions by involving ophthalmologists, general practitioners and ophthalmic nurses. The results showed reasonable inter-observer agreement in assessment. The universal application of the rapid trachoma assessment method is recommended in order to achieve the following:-

i) uniform diagnosis

ii) reproducible recording of diagnosis in studies of prevalence and incidence of trachoma,

iii) evaluating the results of mass antibiotic therapy in the treatment of trachoma

iv) validating the impact of improved environmental conditions.

Mapping of trachoma

The WHO GET Alliance with the support of other WHO agencies and national trachoma control programmes, initiated a very important and interesting project for worldwide mapping of trachoma distribution[1]. The aim of this project is to map countries, regions and areas with high prevalence of active trachoma, trichiasis and entropion (blinding trachoma) as well as with low prevalence of trachoma (non-blinding trachoma). The mapping of trachoma, when completed, may play an important role in planning control programmes by giving priorities to countries, regions, areas and villages with blinding trachoma.

Efficacy of azithromycin

Early studies have shown that a single oral dose of azithromycin is as effective as topical therapy with tetracycline eye ointment applied twice daily for a duration of six weeks[10]. It is also shown that two or three doses of azithromycin given at weekly intervals achieved a cure rate of >90%[10]. The WHO GET Alliance with the support of a pharmaceutical company, and some non-government agencies and national trachoma control programmes in some African countries, initiated a large-scale research project to assess the efficacy of various regimens of azithromycin oral therapy. They also studied logistic problems with regard to supply and distribution of drugs, supervision of treatment at village and family levels, compliance of villagers and adverse effects.

Elimination policy

The WHO GET Alliance has devised a novel and multi-disciplinary strategy for elimination of trachoma by the year 2020. The strategy which is called 'SAFE' consists of:

(S) surgery for entropion and trichiasis

(A) antibiotic therapy

(F) face washing and

(E) environmental improvement

Pilot projects are underway to assess the efficacy of 'SAFE', logistics for application of 'SAFE' strategy, incorporation into existing primary healthcare systems, and materials and human and financial resources required[1].

Surgery
Over 40 surgical techniques are being used for correcting trichiasis and entropion and re-directing lashes away from the cornea[11]. None of these operations provides a lasting result. In some cases, the failure rates may reach up to 20% in the first year and increase substantially in the following years. The WHO GET Alliance presently recommend a bilamellar tarsal rotation procedure which is simple and has a lower failure rate compared with other commonly used operations[1].

It is possible that some ophthalmologists and experts have failed to recognise the fact that surgical procedures are only providing a cosmetic correction. These operations have no influence on the ongoing trachomatous immunopathological processes in the lids. As described earlier, patients with trachoma when re-exposed to CT or its antigenic components, may develop strong cell-mediated responses and delayed hypersensitivity. It is this phenomenon which is responsible for conjunctival scarring, sub-conjunctival and peri-tarsal fibrosis and tarsal degeneration, causing shrinkage and deformity of lids. These immunopathological processes are not affected by lid surgery and will continue and may become exacerbated by further exposure to CT and possibly by operational trauma. In our studies in Iran and Oman, we found that the severity of trachomatous immunopathological processes and the failure rate of lid surgery can be reduced substantially by weekly doxycycline oral therapy for several weeks; and by additional topical therapy with anti-inflammatory drugs.

In most countries with high prevalence of trichiasis and entropion, patients are not enthusiastic towards having corrective lid surgery. Statistics have shown that in some countries (after several years of offering free lid surgery locally or at the nearby hospitals) less than 30% of patients agreed to have the operation.

It might be argued that in order to convince patients with trichiasis and entropion who are already suffering from partial visual defects or who are potentially in danger of losing their sight, to accept surgery, the WHO GET Alliance and national control programmes should base these projects on:

a   an effective health education programme
b   the provision of surgery locally or at nearby hospitals, with

c   free transport for patients and their companions, and free accommodation
      if they have to stay overnight.

Antibiotic therapy
C. trachomatis is sensitive to sulphonamides, tetracyclines, macrolides
(including erythromycin and the newly developed azithromycin), rifamycin
and some quinolones.

Aureomycin eye ointment used twice daily for six weeks is shown to cure
trachoma in up to 70% of cases. However, it was found that intensive and
continuous topical treatment is not practical for the mass therapy of trachoma
in rural communities. As an alternative, the WHO recommended an
intermittent regime with aureomycin eye ointment, twice daily, for five
consecutive days a month for a period of six months per year. The aim of this
method of therapy was to interrupt transmission of CT during the transmission
season, when the fly population is at its greatest and outbreaks of bacterial
conjunctivitis are common. Intermittent therapy with topical antibiotics failed
to reduce prevalence and incidence of trachoma substantially. This failure was
mainly due to inadequate and erratic supply of the antibiotic ointment to the
villages and families, inability of adults to apply eye ointment correctly in to
their own eyes or into the eyes of children and a very low level of compliance.

Azithromycin, a new member of macrolides, is shown to be highly effective
against CT. The minimum inhibitory concentration (MIC) of azithromycin is
shown to be about 0.10–0.25µg per ml[12]. Studies have shown that after a single
oral dose of azithromycin (20mg per kg) the drug can be detected in tears and
serum in concentrations well above its MIC for 96 hours or longer[12]. The
release of azithromycin in body fluids for a long period is due to its high tissue
binding and its slow release from tissues into the blood and other body fluids.

Recent studies on the efficacy of azithromycin oral therapy in hyperendemic
trachoma have shown that a single oral dose of azithromycin (20mg per kg) is as
effective as topical therapy with aureomycin eye ointment applied twice daily
for six weeks. It has also been shown that 2 to 3 oral doses of azithromycin given
at weekly intervals have cured trachoma in up to 90% of patients[10].

Azithromycin oral therapy may provide a highly effective tool for the
elimination of trachoma. However, adoption of azithromycin oral therapy
requires substantial financial resources for purchasing the drug, an efficient
chain of supply and distribution and close supervision.

We are aware that IO International Ltd, a UK based company, is developing
an ocular insert device for sustained and continuous delivery of drugs in the

eye. The results so far have shown that the ocular insert device can be retained in the eye for a period of 3 to 6 months without causing an unacceptable level of irritation and adverse effects. The ocular insert device is capable of continuous release of drugs at a predetermined level and duration. This novel development may provide an opportunity to incorporate azithromycin into the delivery system which would then release the antibiotic continuously for the whole trachoma transmission season. We believe that this concept may provide a much cheaper, more effective and practical alternative to oral therapy.

Face washing
As described earlier, regular face washing of children can remove CT contaminated eye and nasal discharges, hence interrupting the transmission chain of trachoma. To encourage mothers to wash the faces of their children regularly, firstly, there is a need for a supply of clean water accessible to all inhabitants and secondly, a comprehensive and continuing programme of health education.

Environment
It is known that environmental improvements, including improved standards of housing, sanitation and waste disposal have substantial and continuing effects on the prevalence and incidence of trachoma. However, the economic investment required to improve the standard of living and health of trachoma-affected communities may take several years to achieve.

CONCLUSION

While the objective and philosophy of GET by 2020 is of course fully supported, we believe that the above objective may not be achieved without wider specific recognition and subsequently resolution of the following difficulties:

- Magnitude of the problem which involves over 150 million people, spread over 30 countries.
- Inadequate financial, technological, administrative and managerial resources at the national level.
- Lack of political commitment in countries where trachoma is hyperendemic and
- Insufficient financial support by international agencies and industrialised countries to support the WHO GET programme.

We are of the opinion that with resources currently available or which may become available, it is feasible to eliminate blinding trachoma by the year 2020. This would, however, require the following:

a) reducing the prevalence, incidence and severity of trachoma using effective mass antibiotic therapy supplemented by improvement in the standards of hygiene, sanitation and public health,
b) eliminating trichiasis and entropion through the development and application of effective surgical procedures supplemented by chemotherapy to prevent the progress of trachomatous immunopathological processes after surgery, and
c) a comprehensive, sustained and continuing health education programme.

REFERENCES

1. World Health Organization. (1999). *Report of the third meeting of the WHO Alliance for the Global Elimination of Trachoma.* WHO/PBD/GET/99.3.
2. Dwyer RStC, Treharne D, Jones BR *et al.* (1972). Chlamydial infection. Results of micro-immunofluorescence tests for the detection of type-specific antibody in certain Chlamydial infections. *Brit J Vener Dis* **48:** 452–459.
3. Forsey T and Darougar S. (1984). Acute conjunctivitis caused by atypical chlamydial strain: Chlamydia IOL-207. *Brit J Ophthalmology* **68:** 409–411.
4. Darougar S and Jones Barrie R. (1983). Trachoma. *Br Med Bull* **39:** 117–122.
5. Lietman TM, Dawson CR, Osaki SY *et al.* (2000). Clinically active trachoma versus actual chlamydia infection. *MJA* **172:** 93–94.
6. West SK, Rapoza P, Munoz B *et al.* (1991). Epidemiology of ocular chlamydial infection in a trachoma-hyperendemic area. *J Infect Dis* **163:** 752–756.
7. Emerson P, Lindsay SW, Walraven GEL *et al.* (1999). Effect of fly control on trachoma and diarrhoea. *Lancet* **353:** 1401–1403.
8. Schachter J and Dawson CR. (1978). Human chlamydial infecitons. PSG Publishing, Littleton, MA.
9. Thylefors B, Dawson CR, Jones BR *et al.* (1987). A simplified system for the assessment of trachoma and its complications. *Bull World Health Organization* **65:** 477–483.
10. Negrel AD, Marriotts SP. (1998). WHO Alliance for the global elimination of blinding trachoma and the potential use of azithromycin. *Int J Antimicrobial Agents* **10:** 259–262.
11. Reacher MH, Taylor RH. (1990). The management of trachomatous trichiasis. *Rev Int Trachoma* **67:** 233–261.
12. Karcioglu ZA, El-Yazigi A, Jabak MH *et al.* (1998). Pharmacokinetics of azithromycin in Trachoma patients, serum and tear levels. *Ophthalmology* **105:** 658–661.

CHAPTER 12

Chlamydia pneumoniae
and heart disease

Pekka Saikku
Department of Medical Microbiology
University of Oulu, Finland

Chlamydiae are known to cause various heart diseases. Endo-, myo- and pericarditides were associated with chlamydial infections during the first epidemics of psittacosis due to *Chlamydia psittaci*. The commonest Chlamydia of humans, *Chlamydia pneumoniae* has also been incriminated in these disease pictures. Recently, however, greatest attention has been afforded to the association of *C. pneumoniae* with atherosclerosis and coronary heart disease (CHD).

The discovery of disease associations of the chlamydial strain TW-183 in 1985 led to speculation on its ability to cause chronic inflammations typical for other chlamydial species. Since this agent causes about 10% of all pneumonias, its association with chronic obstructive pulmonary disease, asthma and sarcoidosis was in a way natural. Totally unexpected however, was the association of this respiratory agent, now called *C. pneumoniae*, with acute myocardial infarction and chronic coronary heart disease.

The alert came in 1988, when paired serum samples, collected during acute myocardial infarction episodes, showed a seroconversion against an epitope of chlamydial lipopolysaccharide. This seroconversion was lacking in patients with chronic coronary heart disease, but in both patient groups elevated antibody titres against *C. pneumoniae* were found when compared to healthy matched controls. It was suggested that chronic coronary heart disease patients had a chronic *C. pneumoniae* infection and acute myocardial infarction was associated with an acute exacerbation of this infection.

The seroepidemiological association has been verified in numerous studies in many laboratories with different methods of serology. However, antibodies, especially of IgG type, seem to be a marker of atherosclerosis in common and thus have a poor predictive value for cardiac events, which are complications of this extremely prevalent disease condition. IgA antibodies, with their short half-life time, have in some studies been better predictors of future cardiac events. Presence of IgA antibodies can also be a marker of the shift of immune response from the T helper cells type Th1 to Th2, which is not effective against intracellular parasites. Immune complexes have also been used as markers, but their study is difficult and demands expertise. However, the presence of chlamydial proteins in these complexes points to the presence of the agent in the immediate vicinity of coronary circulation. One should always remember that antibodies alone do not show the site of the infection and how active it is. They should be combined with inflammation or autoimmunity markers. More recently, sensitised C-reactive protein measurements and antibodies to heat-shock protein 60 (Hsp60) have been used.

Seroepidemiology cannot prove or disprove a causal association. The next important finding in these studies was the demonstration of the agent directly in atherosclerotic lesions, even in patients without antibodies. There are now over fifty studies, in which the presence of *C. pneumoniae* in atherosclerotic plaques has been shown by electron microscopy, immunohistochemistry, polymerase chain reaction, *in situ* hybridisation and culture. Only rarely has it been found in healthy areas of arteries. The results between different laboratories are variable but about half of the atherosclerotic plaques have been reported to contain *C. pneumoniae* elementary bodies, antigens or nucleic acids. Even claims that all plaques are in fact positive (if studied carefully enough), have been presented. This finding is unique, since among infectious agents only herpes viruses (cytomegalovirus, HSV-1) have sometimes been found in atherosclerotic plaques. *C. pneumoniae* is present in early atherosclerotic lesions and may even be identified in teenagers. Some studies have found the amount of the agent to be greater in advanced plaques or inflamed plaques tending to rupture, but this association has not been uniformly reported.

The problem is: what is this pathogen doing in the plaques? Atherosclerosis is nowadays accepted as an inflammatory condition. Some consider *C. pneumoniae* only as an innocent bystander that has achieved entry into plaques carried within inflammatory cells which have entered the lesion. However, granulomas filled with inflammatory cells only exceptionally show the presence of this agent. Evidence supporting the active participation of *C. pneumoniae* in the inflammatory process is steadily accumulating. *C. pneumoniae* can multiply in the endothelial and smooth muscle cells of the vessel wall and this leads to production of adhesins, cytokines, growth – and tissue factors. A considerable proportion of inflammatory cells extracted from atherosclerotic lesions are targeted against the pathogens present. Macrophages turning to foam cells are the key cells of atherosclerotic lesions. *C. pneumoniae* can multiply in monocytes and macrophages with the respective cytokine induction. Moreover, *C. pneumoniae*-infected macrophages start to ingest low-density-lipoprotein and oxidise it, resulting in formation of foam cells. Some of these reactions can be induced with purified chlamydial components, like lipopolysaccharide (LPS) and chlamydial heat-shock protein 60 (Hsp60). In chronic chlamydial infection, chlamydial Hsp60 is produced in large amounts and it is found in plaques alongside human Hsp60. The continuous presence of chlamydial Hsp60 may eventually lead to autoimmunity against human Hsp60, due to cross-reactive epitopes shared by these highly conserved proteins. According to recent reports, autoimmunity to human Hsp60 seems to be a risk factor for cardiac events. Altogether there seem to be several mechanisms by which *C. pneumoniae* could contribute to the development of atherosclerosis.

Atherosclerosis is a multifactorial disease. There are many risk factors which may be implicated in the pathogenesis. Several risk factors may be associated with chronic *C. pneumoniae* infection or may be partly a reflection of it (**Table 1**). Since the majority of individuals are exposed to *C. pneumoniae* infection during their lifetime, dose, route of infection and genetic factors of

Table 1. Risk factors for coronary heart disease, which have been associated with chronic *C. pneumoniae* infection

A. Affecting the outcome	B. Caused by the infection
– age	– chronic bronchitis
– male gender	– cytokine induction (TNF-alpha, IL-1)
– smoking	– elevation of C-reactive protein
– heredity	– altered lipid profile
– physical activity	– obesity
– diet	– hypertonia
– infections	– fatigue and depression
– stress	– autoimmunity to Hsp60

both the host and the pathogen may determine the final outcome. Some HLA-associations with *C. pneumoniae*-associated CHD have been reported. When *C. pneumoniae* reaches the lungs, it can participate in the development of COPD, a recently recognised risk factor for CHD. Chronic infection leads to elevated cytokine production, which in turn may lead to fatigue and depression, which are also risk factors. Physical activity improves immune defence mechanisms and protects from cardiac events. Chronic *C. pneumoniae* infection is associated with a lipid profile typical for CHD (elevated triglyceride and cholesterol concentrations and lowered high-density-lipoprotein). Markers of inflammation found in atherosclerosis, like C-reactive protein, can be due to chronic *C. pneumoniae* infection. Immune defence mechanisms of smokers are hampered and in our studies on discordant identical twins, the smoking twin had higher IgA antibody levels and lowered cell-mediated immune response against *C. pneumoniae* than the non-smoking twin. Some reports have associated the presence of chronic *C. pneumoniae* with obesity and elevated blood pressure and *C. pneumoniae* also seems to be a factor in the metabolic syndrome.

Animal models are important in the study of atherosclerosis and fortunately several models are available for *C. pneumoniae*. When rabbits are inoculated intranasally by *C. pneumoniae*, those on a normal diet develop atherosclerotic lesions, and in rabbits on a diet enriched with cholesterol, the development of lesions is enhanced. This effect is prevented by macrolides if given early in the disease. *Mycoplasma pneumoniae* given intranasally to rabbits produces a generalised infection, but it does not lead to focal lesions in arteries. In mouse experiments, both normal and gene-knock-out mice have been used. Cholesterol must usually be added in the diet of mice. The development of the atherosclerotic lesions is accelerated by repeated intranasal inoculations of *C. pneumoniae*. Interestingly, *Chlamydia trachomatis* (strain mouse pneumonitis), produces similar systemic infection in mice and can be detected in the aorta after intranasal inoculation. However, it does not persist there and does not cause the development of atherosclerosis. Pigs are also infected and apes are chronically infected with *C. pneumoniae*, but studies on possible atherosclerosis induced in them are lacking.

Bachmeier *et al* (1998) found, when studying mechanisms of viral carditis in mouse, a cross-reactivity of mouse α-actin with the chlamydial major outer membrane protein. A peptide made from this common sequence produced severe carditis associated with coronary thrombi in inoculated mice. They suggested this reaction may be causally related to the association of

Chlamydia with atherosclerosis. However, the cross-reactivity was stronger with MOMP of *C. trachomatis*, which is not associated with atherosclerosis. This cross-reactivity could be of importance in myocarditis and cardiomyopathy. Already in 1974 it was reported that three cases of enterovirus negative carditides in children were due to *C. trachomatis*, and one of these led to cardiomyopathy and death of the patient. These studies have, unfortunately, not been continued.

Final evidence can be found after intervention and vaccination trials. Three small placebo-controlled intervention trials in preventing secondary cardiac events have been published. The first was successful, the second partially successful, and the third inconclusive. At this moment several large intervention trials are going on. The antibiotics used are new macrolides and one fluoroquinolone (**Table 2**). The regimens are variable, treatment can be continuous or intermittent, and the length of treatment may be as long as one year. If these trials are successful, we have immediately a new therapeutic approach to a serious, frequently fatal, disease. The mode of any successful therapeutic reaction would require further evaluation: was some other bacterium treated or was an anti-inflammatory effect responsible for the results (as has been suggested previously)? Three studies on the effect on antibiotic treatment in preventing successive primary cardiac events have been published. One was negative, the other two positive. Markedly, in the study by

Table 2. Some ongoing intervention trials in 2001

Study	No. patients	Antibiotic used	Year completed
WIZARD	7000	Azithromycin for 3 months	2003
ACES	4000	Azithromycin for 1 year	2003
PROVE IT	4000	Gatifloxacin for 18 months	Starts 2000 Follow-up 1.5 years
STAMINA	600	Azithromycin and Helicobacter eradication for 15 days	Follow up 1.5 years
MARBLE	1300	Azithromycin for 3 months	Follow-up 1 year

Meier, the best result was seen after fluoroquinolone treatment (60 per cent protection for three years). Older fluoroquinolones are usually not recommended for acute chlamydial infection. The situation may be altered in chronic chlamydial infections, where protein synthesis could be minimal but nucleic acid synthesis has been reported. Quinolones and rifampicin could be more effective in that situation. According to recent reports, azithromycin treatment alone for *C. pneumoniae* was not successful but in combination with rifampicin, it was effective in eradicating the agent from chronically infected mice. This type of experimentation is essential to ensure that the history of monotherapy in tuberculosis or helicobacter infections does not repeat itself.

The sequencing of the whole genome of *C. pneumoniae* has offered a shortcut for development of candidate vaccines against the pathogen. We do not yet know whether a therapeutic vaccine is either realistic or achievable, but after successful eradication a vaccine should protect from reinfection. Still better, an effective vaccine given in early childhood would be required to afford long-term protection from the development of atherosclerosis, which starts at an early age. However, the final protective effect against acute myocardial infarctions could be seen only some 50 years after administration. The development of other chlamydial vaccines has led to disappointment, short-term/incomplete immunity and the risk of sensitising the recipient.

After initial optimism there have been recent attacks against the role of *C. pneumoniae* in atherosclerosis. Some are based on poorly tested serological methods and fail to understand the nature and individuality of seroresponses. There is no standardised, sensitive commercial PCR test kit for *C. pneumoniae* available. Comparisons of available nucleic acid extraction kits have not been done in sufficient amounts but it is evident that the pathogen is sitting there. However, even if the results of intervention studies are disappointing, the role of *C. pneumoniae* in atherosclerosis is not excluded. This work is clearly not yet complete. Treatment has possibly started too late. Other authors have commented on the disappointing results of late treatment in genital tract infection with *C. trachomatis*. If this is the case then primary intervention studies are needed.

Whilst awaiting the results of ongoing large intervention studies, we should continue animal experiments and studies on pathogenetic mechanisms in order to understand what is going on in *C. pneumoniae* infections. We need to understand the pathogenesis at a subcellular level, in acute, sub-acute and chronic infection.

One should realise that nowadays in both developed and developing countries, cardiovascular diseases are the leading causes of death. Any potential means of alleviating such massive global morbidity and mortality must be thoroughly and fastidiously evaluated.

FURTHER READING

Allegra L, Blasi F (eds). (1999). *Chlamydia pneumoniae.* The Lung and the Heart. 205 pp. Springer Verlag, Milan.

Bachmeier K, Neu N, de la Maza LM, Paö S, Hessel A. Penninger JM. (1999). Chlamydia infections and heart disease linked through antigenic mimicry. *Science* **283**:1335–9.

Campbell LA, Blessing E, Rosenfeld M, Lin TM, Kuo C. (2000). Mouse models of *C. pneumoniae* infection and atherosclerosis. *J Infect Dis.* Jun;**181** Suppl 3:S508–13.

Danesh J, Collins R, Peto R. (1997). Chronic infections and coronary heart disease: is there a link? *Lancet* **350**: 430–6.

Fong IW, Chiu B, Viira E, Jang D, Mahony JB. (1999). De novo induction of atherosclerosis by *Chlamydia pneumoniae* in a rabbit model. *Infect Immun* **67**: 6048–55.

Gupta S, Leatham EW, Carrington D, Mendall MA, Kaski JC, Camm AJ. (1997). Elevated *Chlamydia pneumoniae* antibodies, cardiovascular events, and azithromycin in male survivors of myocardial infarction. *Circulation* **96**: 404–407.

Gurfinkel E, Bozovich G, Beck E, Testa E, Livellara B, Mautner B. (1999). Treatment with the antibiotic roxithromycin in patients with acute non-Q-wave coronary syndromes – The final report of the ROXIS study. *Eur Heart J* **20**: 121–7.

Kalayoglu MV, Hoerneman B, LaVerda D, Morrison SG, Morrison RP, Byrne GI. (1999). Cellular oxidation of low-density lipoprotein by *Chlamydia pneumoniae. J Infect Dis* **180**:780-90.

Kol A, Bourier T, Lichtman AH, Libby P. (1999). Chlamydial and human heat shock protein 60s activate human vascular endothelium, smooth muscle cells, and macrophages. *J Clin Investig* **103**: 571–7.

L'Age-Stehr J (ed). (2000). *Chlamydia pneumoniae* and Chronic Disease. 203 pp.Springer Verlag, Berlin.

Laurila A, Bloigu A, Näyhä S, Hassi J, Leinonen M, Saikku P. (1997). Chronic *Chlamydia pneumoniae* infection is associated with a serum lipid profile known to be a risk factor for atherosclerosis. *Arterioscler Thromb Vasc Biol* **17**: 2910–3.

Leinonen M, Saikku P.(2000). Infections and atherosclerosis. *Scand Cardiovasc J* **34**: 12–20.

Linnanmäki E, Leinonen M, Mattila K, Ekman MR, Nieminen MS, Valtonen V, Saikku P. (1993). Presence of *Chlamydia pneumoniae* specific antibodies in circulating immune complexes in coronary heart disease. *Circulation* **87**: 1130–4.

Maass M, Bartels C, Engel PM, Mamat U, Sievers HH. (1998). Endovascular presence of viable *Chlamydia pneumoniae* is a common phenomenon in coronary artery disease. *J Amer Coll Cardiol* **31**: 827–32.

Mayr M, Kiechl S, Willeit J, Wick G, Xu Q. (2000). Infections, immunity, and atherosclerosis. Association of antibodies to *Chlamydia pneumoniae, Helicobacter pylori,* and cytomegalovirus with immune reactions to heat-shock protein 60 and carotid or femoral atherosclerosis. *Circulation* **102:** 833–9.

Meier CR, Derby LE, Jick SS, Vasilakis C, Jick H. (1999). Antibiotics and risk of subsequent first-time acute myocardial infarction. *JAMA* **281:** 427–31.

Mosorin M, Surcel H-M, Laurila A, Lehtinen M, Karttunen R, Juvonen J, Paavonen J, Morrison RP, Saikku P, Juvonen T. (2000). Detection of *Chlamydia pneumoniae*-reactive T lymphocytes in human atherosclerotic plaques of carotid artery. *Arterioscler Thromb Vasc Biol* **20:** 1061–7.

Muhlestein JB, Anderson JL, Hammond EH, Zhao LP, Trehan S, Schwobe EP, Carlquist JF.(1998). Infection with *Chlamydia pneumoniae* accelerates the development of atherosclerosis and treatment with azithromycin prevents it in a rabbit model. *Circulation* **97:** 633–36.

Ross R. (1999). Atherosclerosis – an inflammatory disease. *N Engl J Med* **340:** 115–26.

CHAPTER 13

Chronic pelvic pain in young women
The importance of differential diagnosis

Richard Beard
Imperial College Medical School, London

Anusha Dias
Northwick Park and St Marks Hospital Trust, Harrow, UK

Pelvic Inflammatory Disease is a very common clinical diagnosis although not so prevalent as a cause of chronic as opposed to acute pelvic pain. This is increasingly supported by detailed microbiological investigation. Twenty year's experience of providing specialist services for women with chronic pelvic pain has clearly established the need for a broadly-based approach to differential diagnosis.

CHRONIC PELVIC PAIN (CPP)

Chronic pelvic pain can be defined as pain that has been present for at least 6 months. In Britain, the prevalence rate has been reported to be 21.5 per 1,000 women which is comparable to the rate of 21.5 for migraine and 41.5 for backache[1]. Davies *et al*[2] found that approximately 350,000 females of reproductive age, suffer from CPP and the complaint accounts for 20% of all gynaecological referrals. Mathias *et al*[3] reported from a Gallup telephone survey of women between the ages of 18-50 years that 14.9 per cent had CPP of sufficient severity for 3 months or more to see their doctors[4]. In 1981, a study found that up to 69% of women with CPP of six months' duration or more had no organic pathology identified at laparoscopy. Although our understanding of CPP has improved in recent years, it is important to remember that non-gynaecological causes (eg abdominal wall pain and bowel pain) can simulate gynaecological pain. Also, CPP that appears to be of gynaecological origin may have causal pathology of organs such as the bladder or large bowel, or even from sites outside the pelvis such as the duodenum, or abdominal wall. It is as well to recognise that visceral pain is an unreliable guide as to the exact site of the somatic cause of the pain.

DYSMENORRHOEA

Dysmenorrhoea is defined as lower abdominal pain occurring around the time of menstruation. It is usually described as a dull ache of variable intensity, and is influenced by various psychosocial and biological factors[5]. Strong positive associations can be demonstrated within families and with early menarche. However, no associations were found with parity and smoking. Several studies have demonstrated the importance of psychological factors. Skandhan et al [6] showed that women with prior knowledge and understanding of menstruation resulted in them having higher rates of menstrual regularity and lower rates of dysmenorrhoea. Gath et al [7] found a high index of neuroticism among dysmenorrhoea sufferers. It is important to distinguish between the two classifications of dysmenorrhoea in current use. The first, primary dysmenorrhoea is defined as pain with no obvious cause, and secondary dysmenorrhoea as pain in the presence of an identified pathology. The practical limitation of this definition is that it assumes that the absence of visible pathology means that the condition is physiological, whereas with secondary dysmenorrhoea it is unreasonably assumed that the visible pathology is certain to be the cause of the pain. Another clinically more useful classification, distinguishes between congestive dysmenorrhoea, which is pain occurring in the late luteal phase of the cycle before the onset often relieved by menstrual flow, and spasmodic dysmenorrhoea which is pain confined to the time of bleeding. The advantage of this definition is that it locates the time in the cycle when the pain occurs without prejudging the cause. Treatment of both congestive and spasmodic dysmenorrhoea is often initially in the form of the combined oral contraceptive pill. If this fails, ovarian steroids and prostaglandin synthetase inhibitors such as mefenamic acid (Ponstan) can be used. Psychological interventions are also helpful[8]. Relaxation training has been found to be effective with spasmodic dysmenorrhoea but not for congestive dysmenorrhoea.

ENDOMETRIOSIS

Endometriosis is an enigmatic disease associated with the presence of endometrium outside the uterine cavity. Its relationship to CPP has been well reviewed by Kennedy and Overton[9]. Roddick *et al* [10] showed that it could present as dysmenorrhoea (45%), deep dysmenorrhoea (16%), rectal pain (8%), as a chronic non-cyclic pelvic ache or be asymptomatic. CPP may also involve other systems such as the gastrointestinal, urinary and pulmonary systems. Within the pelvis, the commonest sites for implantation are the ovary (where it may form chocolate cysts), the peritoneum of the pouch of Douglas, the uterosacral ligaments and the pelvic peritoneum, particularly the broad ligament and uterovesical folds. Ectopic endometrium behaves in the same way as that in the uterus, and it is thought that bleeding in the deposit at the time of menstruation causes a local fibrosis and thus pain.

However there is little correlation between extent of endometriosis and severity of pain[11]. Theories have been postulated to explain why endometriosis causes pain. Some authors feel that retrograde menstruation which is the upward passage of menstrual blood through the fallopian tubes into the pelvic cavity may cause pain. Another theory suggests that reduced mobility of pelvic organs secondary to severe adhesions may be a cause. This could be a result of altered blood flow. The involvement of the autonomic nerves by endometrial tissue may be another possible mechanism. A theory, suggested by Schmidt[12], showed that women with endometriosis had more peritoneal fluid in the pouch of Douglas and that this fluid contained greater quantities of prostaglandin E_2 and $F_{2\alpha}$. These compounds are vasoactive and may cause vascular stasis and therefore pain. Vernon *et al* [13] found that petechial or 'reddish implants' have a greater capacity for synthesising prostaglandin F while black implants have the least capacity. The selection of treatments available for chronic pelvic pain thought to be caused by endometriosis has been well described by Wardle[14]. Options for medical treatment are drugs which suppress ovarian activity to a greater or lesser degree. They include danazol – a derivative of 17α ethinyltestosterone, although this is not much favoured these days because of its androgenising effects. Alternatively, while the GnRH analogues are expensive, they are more effective, better tolerated and without the risk of permanent side effects such as androgenisation. If they are employed, 'add back' therapy (i.e. progesterone with or without oestrogen) should be used to relieve menopausal side-effects and to prevent bone loss[15]. The combined oral contraceptive pill has also been used, as have progestogens such as medroxyprogesterone acetate (Provera). Surgery is the most commonly used treatment for endometriosis. For women who wish to conserve their fertility, this varies from local excision of deposits by open surgery to laparoscopic laser coagulation. For more severe cases, or when fertility is not an issue, total hysterectomy is an option, but this should be accompanied by a bilateral salpingoophorectomy as the growth of endo-metriotic tissue is driven by oestrogens. In young women, removal of the ovaries should be preceded by a 3-4 month period of ovarian down-regulation to ensure that oophorectomy will be effective in curing the pelvic pain.

PELVIC CONGESTION

There is now good evidence to show that 84% of women with an apparently normal pelvis on laparoscopy, have pelvic congestion[16]. The name given to this condition describes the underlying pathophysiology. Inadequate clearance of venous blood results in the release of pain producing substances, the pain experienced being similar to the runner who develops cramp. Much of the study of the condition has been devoted to establishing its existence, so that, to date, the epidemiology of this condition has not been well characterised. However, it does seem likely that it is the cause of most cases that have been classified as 'chronic pelvic pain without obvious pathology' (CPPWOP). Stacey et al [17] reporting on a consecutive series of women investigated laparoscopically for CPP, found that in 60 per cent of them there was no visible pathology. In an audit of clinical activity of a tertiary referral clinic devoted mainly to the investigation of women with CPPWOP over one year, the prevalence of pelvic congestion among 177 women with CPP was 77 per cent (Beard and Rogers unpublished). **Table 1** is a list of all diagnoses and their frequency, found in this audit.

Table 1. Distribution of diagnosis from audit of 177 women who attended a tertiary referral pelvic pain clinic (1997-98)

	n	%
Pelvic congestion	136	77
Ilioinguinal nerve damage	9	5
Trapped ovary(ies)	5	3
Ovarian remnant(s)	2	1
Others – endometriosis, no diagnosis, etc	25	14

Table 2. Frequency of symptoms in two groups with chronic pelvic pain and a normal group of women (Beard *et al*[18])

	Controls (36)	Pelvic Pathology (22)	Pelvic Congestion (35)
Activity-related Pain			
Standing	0%	18%	40%
Walking	0%	18%	49%
Bending/Lifting	0%	9%	60%
Postcoital ache	8%	9%	65%
Deep dyspareunia	11%	41%	71%
Associated Symptoms			
Menorrhagia	22%	27%	54%
Congestive dysmenorrhoea	14%	14%	69%
Spasmodic dysmenorrhoea	36%	59%	9%

DIAGNOSIS OF PELVIC CONGESTION

The most valuable diagnostic indicators of pelvic congestion are the history and clinical findings. **Table 2** is a comparison between symptoms in two groups of women with CPP – those with and without visible pathology at laparoscopy compared with a control group of women without CPP matched for age and parity. Typically, women with pelvic congestion present with a dull and aching pain interspersed occasionally with acute exacerbations. Pain is aggravated by standing, exercise, abdominal straining, intercourse and stress. It is relieved by lying down, relaxation, local heat and analgesics. Sexual problems are common. Of all women with pelvic congestion, 71 per cent complain of dyspareunia and 65 per cent of postcoital ache[18]. This last symptom has a predictive value of 92 per cent for the diagnosis of pelvic congestion. Menstrual cycle defects are common (54%) particularly heavy bleeding in the first two days of menstruation, as is congestive dysmenorrhoea (69%). Women with the condition often complain of vaginal discharge, backache, headache and urinary symptoms and postdefaecation pain (in contrast to the pain of the irritable bowel syndrome when pain is relieved by defaecation).

One of the most important physical signs in the diagnosis of pelvic congestion is ovarian point tenderness, at the junction of the upper and middle one third of a line drawn from umbilicus to anterior superior iliac spine, which is present in 77 per cent of women. Ovarian tenderness is also important, and can be elicited on bimanual examination in 86 per cent of these patients.

Investigations should include a laparoscopy to exclude pelvic inflammatory disease and endometriosis and a vaginal ultrasound scan. Large dilated veins with a congested uterus and/or multicystic ovaries are often seen at laparoscopy and on scan. Adams *et al* [19] and Farquhar *et al* [20] showed with ultrasound scan that 50-56% of women with pelvic congestion have multi- and polycystic ovaries.

Pelvic venogram should be used as an investigative tool if there is any doubt about the cause of chronic pelvic pain – for example when pelvic congestion and endometriosis co-exist.

The transcervical venogram was first described by Topolanski-Sierra in 1958[21]. Beard *et al*[16] have subsequently developed a useful scoring system which quantifies the degree of venous dilation, severity of congestion and clearance of dye with 91 per cent diagnostic sensitivity and 89 per cent specificity. A needle is passed through the cervix to the fundus of the uterus and 20ml of radio-opaque dye is injected into the myometrium. The rate of passage of dye and its rate of clearance through the parauterine, paravesical and ovarian veins and the diameter of the vein, determines whether or not pelvic congestion is present.

PSYCHOLOGICAL FACTORS IN CHRONIC PELVIC PAIN

Psychological factors such as specific attitudes to illness, emotional deprivation in childhood, and physical and sexual abuse are important antecedents for pelvic congestion[22,23] which also make these individuals prone to the adverse effects of stress[24].

The influence of stress on the generation, maintenance, and exacerbation of CPP is shown in **Figure 1**. It illustrates the vicious circle of pain-stress-pain that is present in all individuals that suffer from chronic pain of any sort, but is of particular relevance in functional disorders such as the irritable bowel syndrome and pelvic congestion.

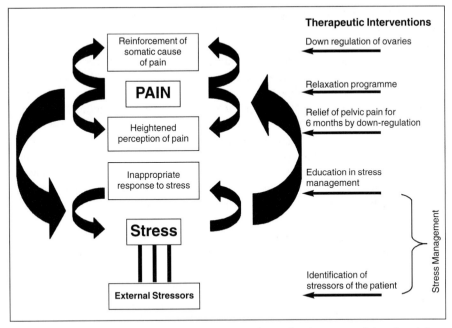

Figure 1. Explanatory scheme to explain the generation and maintenance of chronic pelvic pain and treatment

TREATMENT

The aim of treatment is to return women to an acceptable quality of life by teaching them that they are able to control and often to eliminate their pelvic pain. This is achieved by using medical therapy to induce a pain-free interval of approximately six months during which time, women, after psychological assessment, are taught stress and pain management. A variety of treatment programmes are described in *The Textbook of Pain*[25]. The place of specific interventions in relation to the psychological factors are shown graphically in **Figure 1**. It is important to reassure these women from the outset of treatment that the correct diagnosis has been made by inducing a relatively pain-free time in their lives with one of the GnRH analogues to achieve complete ovarian down regulation. Experience has shown that this is most effective in women who become amenorrhoeic on this treatment. Menopausal symptoms, which may be quite disabling in some women, can be effectively treated by the use of add-back HRT throughout the period of ovarian down regulation. It is important to ensure that whilst the patient is on medical therapy, she is concurrently receiving formal stress and pain management counselling. Pearce *et al*[24] showed an increase in the number of pain-free days in women who received counselling in the clinic setting who were taught relaxation techniques. We have found that those patients who actively avoid the counselling, are most likely to complain of continued CPP and breakthrough bleeding whilst on down regulation. Once they have completed treatment, these women are least likely to be able to control the CPP when their menses are resumed. When medical therapy comes to an end, the patient should be ready to apply the lessons she has learnt in the counselling sessions. Quite simply, this involves a progressive reduction in stressful activities such as emotionally or physically demanding jobs, applying techniques they have learnt on how to handle stress in a more appropriate manner, and whenever an attack of pain is starting, the use of relaxation techniques they have learnt . In 70-75 per cent of patients the cause of their pain is understood and no longer dominates their lives. They find that they have learnt what brings on the pain and they can control it. In other words, they no longer fear the pain, and as the attacks of pain diminish in severity, so the quality of their lives improves. For most, they find, within a year of starting treatment that CPP is no longer a problem in their lives. The great value of this conservative approach to treatment is that young women are able to return to a normal life without having had to compromise ovarian function.

Removal of the ovaries combined with hysterectomy remains a last resort for a few women. Beard *et al* [26] found that of 778 women referred to the Pelvic Pain Clinic, only 36 of them were suitable for a total hysterectomy and bilateral salpingoophorectomy (TAH and BSO). Most of these women were living in highly stressful situations and found that although they had become pain free on ovarian down-regulation, the CPP had returned with the same intensity after coming off treatment. The operation is highly effective, as is shown by the fact that one year after surgery, 33 of the women were pain free, and all were well established on a satisfactory HRT regimen. In summary, it is our experience that there is a small group of women of reproductive age, with CPP, whose quality of life is so poor that surgical removal of their ovaries is justified.

THE CASE FOR BILATERAL OOPHORECTOMY IN YOUNG WOMEN

Most gynaecologists believe that ovarian function should always be conserved in women under the age of 40, except when an ovary is malignant. This view has historical origins from the end of the nineteenth century when ovaries were increasingly being removed unnecessarily from young women. However, there is now an increasing body of evidence that conservation of the ovaries in women of reproductive age 'at all costs' is not always justified[27,28].

Ovaries which are apparently normal histologically may give rise to a number of symptoms such as chronic pelvic pain and/or severe cyclical premenstrual tension. If sufficiently severe, these symptoms may seriously interfere with the quality of life of women at a time in their lives when they are least likely to tolerate any impairment of their daily living. In a review of five women under the age of 35 years after they had had a bilateral oophorectomy for one of the above conditions by Carey[29], none of them regretted their decision. The only complaint of two of them was that if they had had the operation earlier, they would not have wasted so much of their lives when they most wanted to be free of any impairment. Mention has already been made of the study in which both ovaries were removed from 36 women with a mean age of 30 years as the only effective way of giving them relief from unremitting pelvic pain[26]. The point has to be made that the decision to do the operation was finally made by the patient and her partner and at no time was subsequently regretted. The benefit to 33 of the women was that they became pain free, resulting in a return to a normal quality of life that they had not believed possible. The authors stressed the need for careful selection and counselling of such women before undertaking such an operation, but the reality is that many sensible women in the same situation would have asked for the operation much earlier in their lives.

CHRONIC PELVIC INFLAMMATORY DISEASE (PID)

Although chlamydial PID is described in detail in Chapter 8, a brief gynaecological overview merits consideration.

Chronic PID is a consequence of acute pelvic infection which may lead to permanent damage to the fallopian tubes. The effect of resultant adhesions on the surrounding pelvic organs is variable. In most cases they do not affect the mobility of the uterus, appendages or bowel - if they do, this may give rise to pelvic pain, particularly if the ovaries are involved (see "trapped ovaries"). Chronic PID describes a clinical condition, which may include an intermittent or continuous pelvic pain, but is usually asymptomatic. Although women with recurrent pelvic pain are often diagnosed as having chronic PID, there is no good published evidence that they are having repeated pelvic infections. Young women who present with an acute attack of lower abdominal pain are treated on the presumption that they have acute salpingitis, after which as further attacks of pain occur, it is a short step for them to be labelled as having 'chronic PID', with all the negative associations that such a diagnosis carries. PID is often a diagnosis made without adequate investigation. Stacey *et al*[17] showed that in 40 per cent of women presenting with an attack of acute pelvic pain, the pelvis was normal, at laparoscopy. Conversely, women with laparoscopic evidence of chronic PID do not necessarily give a history of acute PID – for example chlamydial salpingitis is frequently asymptomatic. If the diagnosis of PID is clearcut with lower abdominal pain, pyrexia and a heavy infected vaginal discharge, then treatment with antibiotics is appropriate without resorting to laparoscopy. If, however, this clinical presentation is not present or the pain recurs after adequate antibiotic treatment then a full investigation which includes laparoscopy, pelvic ultrasound, and pelvic venography should be undertaken before a definitive diagnosis is made.

RESIDUAL AND TRAPPED OVARIES

Peritoneal adhesions are usually asymptomatic but can cause pain if they are extensive particularly if they encapsulate an ovary, creating a 'trapped ovary'[30,31]. Surgical removal of the ovaries is the most effective way of relieving the CPP, but adhesiolysis is sometimes as effective but with the added risk of reformation of the adhesions with the return of the pain.

OVARIAN REMNANT SYNDROME

In this condition, fragments of ovary are left behind following what is frequently a difficult oophorectomy. These remnants may become active, often after 1-2 years of quiescence[30]. Typically women present with constant or cyclical pain on one or other side of the pelvis. Postcoital ache and pain after defaecation or micturition, is common. Localised tenderness can be elicited per abdomen even though there are no masses that can be felt on vaginal examination. Serum gonadotrophin concentrations are usually in the premenopausal range and are a useful diagnostic indicator. Ultrasound scanning is critical. Optimal treatment is by surgical removal of the ovarian remnant. Finding the remnant at laparotomy is enhanced by pre-treatment of the women with tabs (clomiphene 50mg daily for ten days), when there may be a concomitant increase in the severity of the pelvic pain which is a further useful diagnostic symptom.

VULVODYNIA

This is a severe intractable burning pain most commonly presenting in postmenopausal women which, contrary to pelvic congestion, is made worse by lying down and better by walking around. While the aetiology is unknown, it is likely to be due to a disturbance by control of the local circulation. History reveals the site of pain being more perineal than vaginal. Examination is unremarkable apart from some perineal or levator ani muscle tenderness. To date, no effective treatment exists for this distressing condition.

ILIOINGUINAL NERVE ENTRAPMENT SYNDROME

This is a relatively common cause of chronic pelvic pain, presentation of which mimics pelvic congestion. The ilioinguinal nerve originates from L1 and L2, runs forwards along the ilium from its dorsal origin to the ventral surface, passes through the abdominal muscle 1–2cm medial to the anterior superior iliac spine and emerges to supply the skin over the mons pubis, vulva, and front of the upper thigh. It can be compressed as it emerges through the muscles or more commonly damaged by operations in this region such as the Pfannenstiel and McBurney incisions. Typically the pain is aching and made worse by any whole body exercise, including sexual intercourse. Tenderness is increased by pressing on a point 1–2cm medial to the anterior superior iliac spine when the patient has been asked to tense her abdominal muscles. The diagnosis is confirmed by relief of the pain for 6–8 hours following injection of 10–20ml of 0.5% bupivicaine around the course of the nerve. Division of the nerve transabdominally is an easy operation which is also the most effective way of relieving a pain that has often been present for many years[32].

IRRITABLE BOWEL SYNDROME (IBS)

This is a common non-gynaecological functional (psychosomatic) disturbance of the large bowel presenting with colicky abdominal pain with abdominal bloating and a bowel habit alternating between the passage of loose stools with mucus and constipation. Sufferers are polysymptomatic and have been found to be over anxious and highly sensitive[33]. Although IBS can simulate pelvic congestion, with pelvic pain, bloating and deep dyspareunia as shared symptoms, bowel dysfunction tends to predominate in the former[34]. A combination of debulking agents and psychotherapy has been shown by Svedlund *et al*[35] to be the most effective treatment.

CONCLUSION

In summary, there are many conditions, both gynaecological and non-gynaecological, which can cause CPP. However, it cannot be overemphasised that in most cases the diagnosis can usually be made on a careful history and physical examination. The authors have found that a structured questionnaire which the patient completes before coming to the clinic is a good way of obtaining most of the information required and for making an initial contact with the patient. Laparoscopy with photographs and a vaginal ultrasound scan are also useful for providing patients with graphic evidence that helps them to understand the diagnosis. Finally, ready resort to asking for advice from colleagues in relevant specialities is an important part of the investigation and treatment of women with CPP. Treatment must be multidisciplinary and involve medical, surgical and psychological approaches.

REFERENCES

1. Zondervan KT Yudkin PL, Vessey MP *et al.*(1999) Prevalence and incidence of chronic pelvic pain in primary care: evidence from a national general practice database *Brit J Obstet Gynaecol* **106:** 1149–1155
2. Davies L, Gangar KF, Drummond MS, *et al.* (1992). The economic burden of intractable gynaecological pain. *J Obstet Gynaecol* **12** (suppl 2); 54–56.
3. Matthias SD, Kupperman M. Liberman R, *et al.* (1996) Chronic pelvic pain; prevalence, health related quality of life and economic correlates. *Obstet Gyaecol* **87:** 321–7.
4. Gillibrand P (1981). The investigation of pelvic pain. Communication at the Scientific Meeting at the Royal College of Obstetrics and Gynaecology, London.
5. Andersch B, Milsom I. (1982). An epidemiologic study of young women with dysmenorrhoea. *Am. J Obstet Gynecol* **44:** 655–660.
6. Skandham KP, Pandya AK, Skandhaus, *et al.*(1988). Menarche: prior knowledge and experience. *Adolescence* **23:** 149–154

7. Gath D, Osbourn M, Burgany G *et al.*(1987). Psychiatric disorder and gynaecological symptoms in middle-aged women. A community survey *Brit Med J* **294:** 213–218
8. Chesney M, Tasto D. (1975). The effectiveness of behaviour modification with spasmodic and congestive dysmenorrhoea. *Behaviour Research and Therapy* **19:** 303–313
9. Kennedy S, Overton C. (1993). Endometriosis and pelvic pain. *Contemp Rev Obstet Gynaecol* **5:** 94–97.
10. Roddick JW, Conkey G, Jacobs EJ (1960). The hormonal response of endometrium in endometriotic implants and its relationship to symptomatology. *Am J Obstet Gynaecol* **79:** 1173–1177
11. Ling (1999). Randomized controlled trial of depot leuprolide in patients with chronic pelvic pain and clinically suspected endometriosis. *Obstet Gynecol*. **93:**
12. Schmidt C (1985). Endometrium: a reappraisal of pathogenesis and treatment. *Fertil Steril* **44:** 157–173.
13. Vernon MW, Beard JS, Graves K, *et al* . (1986). Classification of endometriotic implants by morphological appearance and capacity to synthesize prostaglandin F. *Fertil Steril* **46:** 801–805.
14. Wardle P (1992). In: Shaw RW ed. Conference Report: Intractable gynaecological pain – new management strategies. Royal College of Obstetricians and Gynaecologists, 1 April 1992. *Brit J Obstet Gynaecol* **12:** 355–359.
15. Royal College of Obstetricians and Gynaecologists, The investigation and management of endometriosis.Guidelines No. 24, July 2000
16. Beard RW, Hyman JW, Pearce S, *et al.* (1984). Diagnosis of pelvic varicosities in women with chronic pelvic pain. *Lancet* **ii:** 946–949
17. Stacey CM, Munday PE, Beard RW (1989). Pelvic inflammatory disease, diagnosis and microbiology. Presented at Silver Jubilee Congress of Obstetrics & Gynaecology, London July 1989
18. Beard RW, Reginald PW, Wadsworth J (1988). Clinical features of women with chronic lower abdominal pain and pelvic congestion. *Brit J Obstet Gynaecol* **95:** 153–161.
19. Adams J, Reginald PW, Franks S *et al.* (1990). Uterine size and endometrial thickness and the significance of cystic ovaries in women with pelvic pain due to congestion. *Br J of Obstet Gynaecol* **97:** 583–587
20. Farquhar CM, Rogers V, Franks S, *et al.* (1989). A randomised controlled trial of medoxyprogesterone acetate and psychotherapy for the treatment of pelvic congestion. *Br J Obstet Gynaecol* **96:** 1153–1162.
21. Topolanski-Sierra R. (1958). Pelvic phlebotgraphy. *Am J Obstet Gynecol* **67:** 44–52
22. Fry RPW, Beard RW,Crisp AH, *et al.* (1997) Sociopsychological factors in women with and without chronic pelvic venous congestion *J Psychosom Res* **42:** 71–85
23. Reiter RC (1990). A profile of women with chronic pelvic pain. *Clin Obstet Gynecol* **33:** 130–136
24. Pearce S, Knight C, Beard RW. (1982). Pelvic pain – a common gynaecological problem. *J Psychosom Obstet Gynaecol* **1:** 12–17
25. Beard RW, Gangar KF, Pearce S. (1994). In. Wall PW, Melzack R editors. Gynaecological Pain. Textbook of Pain. Churchill Livingstone Edinburgh p.597–814.
26. Beard RW, Kennedy RG, Gangar KF. (1991). Bilateral oophorectomy and hysterectomy in the treatment of intractable pelvic pain with pelvic congestion. *Br J Obstet Gynaecol* **98:** 988–992
27. Reid BA, Gangar KF, Rogers V. *et al.* (1996). Long term results of bilateral oophorectomy for the treatment of chronic pelvic pain: relief of pain and special hormone replacement therapy requirements *J Obstet Gynaecol* **16:** 538–543
28. Casson P, Hahn PM,Van Vugt DA and Reid RL. (1990). Lasting response to ovariectomy in severe intractable premenstrual syndrome. *Am J Obstet Gynecol* **162:** 99–105
29. Carey A.(1997). Proc. Fed.Int.Gynec.Obstet. Congress, Copenhagen
30. Siddall-Allum J, Witherow R, Beard RW. (1994). Chronic pelvic pain caused by residual ovaries and ovarian remnants. *Br J Obstet Gynaecol* **101:** 979–985.

31. Christ JL, Lotze EC. (1975). The residual ovary syndrome. *Obstet Gynecol* **46:** 555–556.
32. Hahn L (1989). Clinical findings and results of operative treatment in ilioinguinal nerve entrapment syndrome. *Br J Obstet Gynaecol.* **96:** 1080–1083
33. Heaton KW (1983). Irritable bowel syndrome: still in search of its identity. *Br Med J* **287:** 852–853
34. Farquhar CM, Hoghton GBS, Beard RW. (1990). Pelvic pain – pelvic congestion or the irritable bowel syndrome? *Europ J Obstet Gynaecol and Reprod Biol* **37:** 71–75
35. Svedlund J, Ottoson J-O, Sjodin I, *et al.* (l983). Controlled study of psychotherapy in irritable bowel syndrome. *Lancet* **ii:** 589–592

CHAPTER 14

Chlamydial infections – an overview
Is it time for a wider/broader hypothesis?

Robert S Morton
Sheffield, UK

INTRODUCTION

The genus Chlamydia may be listed as follows:

1. *C. trachomatis* with its serovars A, B, B1 and C, the cause of trachoma, the commonest cause of early blindness in the third world; its serovars D to K the cause of an increasingly common genito-urinary infection with chronic and costly complications in perhaps 10 per cent; and its serovars L1, L2 and L3 the cause of lymphogranuloma venereum, now a relatively rare form of sexually transmitted disease with occasionally crippling complications.

2. *C. psittaci*, the cause of a rare form of chest infection in humans and birds particularly.

3. *C. pneumoniae*, the cause of acute pulmonary infections in humans in the western world. In some it has chronic, crippling and killing complications. Neither its prevalence nor morbidity rate have been adequately defined.

In the last half century it has become clear that while antibiotics effect clinical cure in these infections, they do not appear to eradicate the organism in many cases. In psitticosis, apparently cured humans and birds may continue to excrete organisms. In other chlamydial diseases relapses are regularly recognised. In all of the chlamydial infections listed asymptomatic periods of months or years may be followed by emergence of late overt disease.

Thus chlamydial infections can be viewed as having three stages – early, latent and late.

PATHOGENESIS OF CHLAMYDIAL INFECTIONS

Early chlamydial disease begins with serial infection of surface epithelial cells. This is effected by receptor-mediated endocytosis. Once inside a cell Chlamydiae are contained within host derived endosomes. They coalesce within these cytoplasmic vacuoles. By utilising cellular material these ingested elementary bodies (EB) metamorphose into reticulate bodies (RB).

These undergo binary fission, mature and are released as EB on the natural death of the infected epithelial cell. The life cycle takes between 48 and 72 hours.

Dying epithelial cells also release cytokines[1] which prompt increased blood supply and increased permeability of basal membranes. Together these allow migration of lymph node cells, diapedesing from venules to reach the infected area and phagocytose invading and shed Chlamydiae. In 1989 Shahmanesh[2] described the distinctive differential white cell count associated with acute chlamydial urethritis in men (**Table 1**). At the same time Chlamydiae travel to the relevant lymph nodes. In some cases of urethritis they can be demonstrated by culture of lymph gland puncture material.

Table 1. Percentage of different inflammatory cells in urethral exudants from men with non-gonococcal urethritis (NGU) for the first time, presumed re-infections and recurrences without known sexual re-exposure.

Cells	First NGU (n = 18)	"Re-infections" (n = 19)	Other Recurrencies (n= 19)
Macrophages	8.5 (5.4)*	2.0 (1.5)	2.3 (1.7)
Lymphocytes	2.6 (2.6)	1.6 (1.8)	1.6 (1.3)
Polymorphs	89 (7.0)	96.3 (2.3)	97.2 (2.33)

* n < 0.01 compared with both other groups.

Figures are mean (SD) obtained from May-Grünweld-Giemsa and Papanicolaou smears.

Complete phagocytosis is accomplished mainly by neutrophils. In addition to phagocytosis lymphocytes play a variety of roles, not least producing gamma interferons (IFN-Ý)[3] which amongst other functions improve the ability of monocytes and macrophages to ingest Chlamydiae. There is some evidence that IFN-Ý, depending on concentration, may play a role in Chlamydia persistence and reactivation.

Immune responses vary in degree between the chlamydial infections. Cellular responses predominate in trachoma and genitourinary disease. Serological responses are recognised only in *C. pneumoniae* disease and in lymphogranuloma venereum. Research on this aspect regarding responses to *C. trachomatis*, serovars D-K continues.

In the late stages of chlamydial infections cellular immune responses are generally described as delayed hypersensitivity. It manifests leucocytes, lymphoid follicles, plasma cell infiltrations, fibroblasts and macrophages. In terms of clearing or containing antigenic material these responses are effective. But this occurs at a price. Extensive fibrosis produces paradoxical healing. Hence the blindness of trachoma, the pelvic scarring in lymphogranuloma venereum, the bone, joint, fascia and crippling scarring of fallopian tubes in genitourinary disease and of no less importance; the chronic, crippling and killing cardiovascular late forms of *C. pneumoniae* infections[4,5].

EARLY FORMS OF CHLAMYDIAL INFECTIONS

Trachoma presents as a persistent acute, bilateral conjunctivitis. Lymphogranuloma venereum, by contrast, presents as an evanescent genital sore lasting only a few days when the disease is then manifest in inguinal and pelvic glands. *C. psittaci* and *C. pneumoniae* both cause acute respiratory disease such as bronchopneumonia or pneumonia. Early genitourinary disease in men presents as acute anterior urethritis with discharge varying from the slight mucoid to the profuse purulent. In females, endocervicitis, with or without symptoms and a variable degree of discharge is usual. Urethritis may also occur in females. Proctitis may affect both sexes.

DIAGNOSIS

In the case of trachoma clinical diagnosis may be confirmed by culture or more modern tests. Nature's ability to clear antigenic material is thought to depend on the original organismal load and its duration. T. cell responses are depressed in persistent trachoma. Diagnosis of lymphogranuloma venereum generally calls for laboratory testing of inguinal lymph gland material and perhaps more than one lymphogranuloma venereum complement fixation test (LGVCFT).

The serological test for *C. pneumoniae* infection is commonly deployed in departments dealing with infectious diseases. So far as can be gathered it is more commonly used in cardiovascular departments in Scandinavia than elsewhere. In Finland *C. pneumoniae's* role in atheroma[6], in degenerative aortic stenosis[7] and in infra-renal aneurysms[8] has been defined.

It is in the genitourinary infections that laboratory tests for Chlamydiae have been most thoroughly developed. From culture and monoclonal antibody testing, progress has been through polymerase and ligase chain reactions to a transcription mediated amplification test as the new gold standard. Thus reliable testing can now be applied to urine and self-taken genital swabs. In so-called first attacks of non-gonococcal urethritis *C. trachomatis* can be identified in around 70 per cent. These modern tests have revealed that some symptomless and signless patients may be carriers. There is in such cases, need for careful history taking and clinical examinations that aim to exclude asymptomatic complications such as prostatitis and salpingitis.

COMPLICATIONS OF TRACHOMA

Systemic complications of trachoma are virtually unknown. This contrasts with ophthalmia neonatorum due to *C. trachomatis* serovars D-K where pneumonia is recognised as an occasional complication. Joint and neurological complications are associated with serovars L1, L2 and L3. Application of the LGVCFT in a West Indian female with idiopathic multiple arthritis proved revealing. The persistent excretion of *C. psittaci* in "cured" humans and birds has led to destruction of exotic birds and closure of public aviaries.

In genitourinary disease, contiguous spread is common. In men, spread to the posterior urethra may be followed by chronic prostatitis or acute unilateral epididymitis. Only recently has *C. trachomatis* been found in prostatic material and then only in 4 of 135 cases[9]. In epididymitis the organism can be found in needle puncture specimens of the affected organ. Canalicular spread from the endocervix is common. As many as 10 per cent of infected women may suffer from endometritis followed by acute, subacute or chronic asymptomatic salpingitis. Recurrent acute and subacute attacks are recognised. Between 1 and 2 per cent of men with NGU develop Reiter's syndrome, partial or complete, with multiple arthritis, conjunctivitis or iritis and skin lesions. All of these have revealed *C. trachomatis* or its antigenic remnants[10,11]. Another[12,13] early complication is Fitz-Hugh–Curtis syndrome which consists of acute peritonitis and peri-hepatitis with a variable degree of ascites. It can occur without evidence of pelvic infection. That the syndrome is due to *C. trachomatis* was described by Shanahan in 1990[14]. With the organisms he cultured in specimens from humans he gave mice peritonitis. He subsequently "cured" both humans and mice without surgery, that is, with antibiotics only. At follow-up Shanahan found Chlamydiae in the spleens of both "cured" humans and mice.

TREATMENT OF EARLY CHLAMYDIAL INFECTIONS

Antibiotics have been effectively applied to all forms, generally for a week or longer in uncomplicated cases and up to three weeks or longer in complicated cases. The application of a wide variety of antibiotics has been well-documented in men with non-gonococcal urethritis. From the early 1950s to the late 1980s these effected high "cure" rates as estimated by clinical follow-up for three months. In the last decade a single dose treatment with azithromycin has become increasingly popular. Follow-up in these cases has been by laboratory testing after four weeks. One study found positive polymerase chain reaction tests in 5 of 98 females[15].

RECURRENT EARLY INFECTION

Early recurrence is well-recognised in all forms of chlamydial disease. It is seen as relapse and this applies to both treated humans and laboratory infected animals.

In lymphogranuloma venereum suspected relapses can generally be confirmed by rising titres of the LGVCFT. In recurrences of trachoma the relevant serovars are rarely detected. It is otherwise in suspected recurrences of chlamydial pneumonia. One report found the organism in 19 of 24 such cases[16].

Recurrence rates of NGU in the 1950s to 1980s were generally above 15 per cent at three months follow-up. Of 221 cases followed up by Munday for a year, recurrence occurred in 45 (20 per cent)[17], A three year follow-up of treated females showed a 38 per cent recurrence rate[18]. Little wonder then that one clinician who followed treated males for 5 years declared "Treatment helps – but not much." (Fowler, personal communication.)

In the last decade, after a single dose of azithromycin, application of the polymerase chain reaction to 98 females gave positive results in 5 (5.1 per cent)[15]. Three months clinical follow-up in similarly treated males gave a recurrence rate of 12 per cent[19]. One attempt to minimise recurrences of NGU compared results of triple tetracycline given for one and three weeks. The recurrence rate at three months was halved[20].

Hurst *et al.* treated groups of mice infected peritoneally with the organisms of lymphogranuloma venereum, psittacosis and trachoma for 200 consecutive days. This eliminated recurrences. At post mortem he found Chlamydiae in spleens and livers[21-23].

THE NATURE OF RECURRENCES

Only in NGU is the nature of recurrences questioned. Some clinicians see such cases as re-infections even when re-exposure has been denied. That recurrences are more likely to be relapses is supported by a variety of clinical observations. Firstly, the sexual histories given by the men contrasts with those given by men with recurrence of gonorrhoea. Evans has given details[24]. Second, are the findings of Hurst *et al.* (*vide supra*) and thirdly, four out of six studies show that treatment of sex partners does not influence recurrence rates of NGU in men[25-30].

A persistent and striking feature of recurrences of NGU is that yields of positive diagnostic tests for *C. trachomatis* are usually half those found in initial attacks, for example, 35 per cent as against 70 per cent. Shamanesh *et al.* in 1996[31] reported the accompanying differential white cell counts in initial and recurrent episodes in both Chlamydia positive and Chlamydia negative cases. The lowest lymphocyte counts were in Chlamydia negative recurrences. It is a well-established truism that re-infection with an organism previously subjected to primary immune responses is more assertively, more speedily and hence more effectively dealt with by a secondary immune response. This is attributed to the establishment of memory, helper and killer cells as part of the primary immune response. The poor yield of positive tests for *C. trachomatis* in recurrences can be seen as nature's success.

Does it matter whether recurrences originate exogenously or endogenously? This question is prompted by the observation that positive tests for *C. trachomatis* are more common in men with gonorrhoea than in men with NGU. Formerly, prompt treatment and cure of gonorrhoea was followed after some days by post-gonococcal NGU. This was clinically acceptable; it reflected differing incubation periods. In modern times, tests for both the gonococcus and the *C. trachomatis* are carried out at the initial attendance. Commonly both are found positive. Presumably some men have been carriers (*vide supra*) and others are incubating, one of two concomitantly acquired diseases. Could there be a third reason? Is it possible that the gonococcus has unmasked latent chlamydial infection? We know that any form of urethritis can reveal asymptomatic HIV infection, a condition in which some 80 per cent of the organismal load exists in the lymphatic system[32,33].

This explanation can be extended to explain why bacillary dysentery may precipitate Reiter's syndrome. It is noteworthy that dual infections are said to account for the observation that recurrences of PID respond better to combined treatment by an antibiotic and metronidazole. The same treatment approach has been useful in recurrent chlamydial chest infections[34].

There seems to be little doubt that a latent stage is a serious reality in some chlamydial infections. Before trying to define its nature let us look at the late overt stages.

LATE OVERT DISEASE

The course of late complications usually follows a long period of surreptitious and often symptomless and signless progress. Trachoma ends with blindness due to chronic low grade infection and scarring. In lympho-granuloma venereum the lower bowel is involved in the progressive scarring of lymph channels. "Pencil" stools result. In women progressive and recurrent episodes of pelvic infection due to serovars D-K commonly produce scarring that results in ectopic pregnancies and sterility. In men bone, joint and fascial deformities are common. Host genetics such as the Class 1 allele HLA-A31 and HLA-B27 may be associated in females and males respectively.

Late cardiovascular and pulmonary complications of *C. pneumoniae* infection have recently been described. The organism is frequently present in arthromatous plaques[4], in cases of degenerative aortic stenosis[7] and in infra-renal abdominal aortic aneurysms[8]. All such cases were also positive by the specific serological test for *C. pneumoniae* infection[4,7,8]. It is of interest to note that while antibiotics as well as immune responses may succeed in effecting some degree of clinical cure by reducing the organismal load in early overt disease, neither is as effective a feature in the late stages[35,36]. This is particularly so in *C. pneumoniae* infections. Even when antibiotics have been taken for a year there is little or no apparent benefit[37]. Chronic and continuous cardiovascular disease activity persists and proves to be both crippling and killing.

THE NATURE OF LATENT CHLAMYDIAL INFECTIONS

From what we know, the most likely siting for latent chlamydial infection is the lymphatic system, including the spleen. If this is true, how are Chlamydiae held in a state of suspended animation for months or years? How do these organisms remain capable of maintaining continuous pathological activity elsewhere for long periods? How are Chlamydiae transported to precipitate early and late overt complications?

It is suggested that the work of Shahmanesh *et al* in 1996 gives a clue. They accorded a dominant role to macrophages in all forms of immune cellular responses to Chlamydiae. Macrophages are descendants of monocytes which are capable of harbouring Chlamydiae for 10 days. Macrophages are also capable of harbouring Chlamydiae and they have a life cycle of a month. Macrophages also circulate freely, some taking up residence in spleen, lungs and serous cavities as well as lymph nodes. They are attracted to sites of inflammation. They are recognised as persisting in inguinal and pelvic glands in lymphogranuloma venereum. Their presence in abundance has been noted in early *C. pneumoniae* infections[38].

From the abundance of clinical observations now available it has recently been hypothesised that macrophages parasitise Chlamydiae. This truncated state of phagocytosis appears to protect the organisms from both immune responses and antibiotics. The effect of both is confined to action only on the death of each macrophage and the shedding of EB and before they can be ingested by a new generation of macrophages. This serial process maintains latency and no less a low grade but progressive late disease process which ends in overt manifestations. The accompanying bio-chemical or molecular responses which support the hypothesis are detailed[39].

Thus all chlamydial diseases may be seen as having three stages – early, latent or late. In many, late manifestations result from years of persistent, low grade but progressive 'delayed hypersensitivity' ending with paradoxical healing causing chronic, crippling or in some, killing end results. There are memories here of syphilis.

THE FUTURE

Lymphogranuloma venereum and psittacosis are currently well controlled. Trachoma prevalence diminishes where running water and improved personal hygiene are made available. The World Health Organisation plans to eliminate trachoma by the year 2020. The plan will utilise a donation of azithromycin by Pfizer valued at £41 million.

In the UK we are about to introduce a nationwide screening programme to detect *C. trachomatis* serovars D-K. The emphasis is on prevention by early diagnosis and treatment of both index cases and their contacts. Consideration regarding which of the infected should be held in long term follow-up remains to be determined. Family histories may indicate those genetically predisposed to late overt disease: HLA studies should be considered. Those presenting with idiopathic iritis and found to have chronic prostatitis and/or sacro-ileitis should be considered as should all cases of salpingitis. Annual review of cases of Reiter's syndrome is already a standard procedure in some departments of genitourinary medicine.

While genitourinary chlamydial disease is believed to cost the UK £50 million per annum, no such estimate is available for *C. pneumoniae* infection. Its chronic, crippling and killing process is unlikely to cost less. Consideration of a preventive approach is indicated. There appears to be potential in the availability of a serological test for this chlamydial condition from an early stage. Its application to young people, that is, at a time when antibiotics may be effective, offers a chance to prevent cardiovascular complications. Widespread serological testing for syphilis in the 20th century was both health and wealth promoting.

REFERENCES

1. Rasmussen SJ, Eckmann I, Quayle AJ, *et al.* (1997). Secretion of proinflammatory cytokines by epithelial cells in response to chlamydial infection suggests a central role for epithelial cells in chlamydial pathogenesis. *J Clin Invest* **99:** 77–87.
2. Shahmanesh M. (1989). Characteristics of inflammatory cells in urethral smears from men with non-gonococcal urethritis. *Genitourin Med* **65:** 18–21.
3. Lampe MF, Wilson CB, Bevan MJ and Starnbach MN. (1998). Gamma interferon production by cytotoxic T lymphocytes as required for resolution of *Chlamydia trachomatis* infection. *Infect Immun* **66:** 5457–61.
4. Mendall MA, Carrington D, Strachan D *et al.* (1995). *Chlamydia pneumoniae*: risk factors for seropositivity and association with coronary heart disease. *Infect* **30:** 121–8.
5. Saikku P, Matilla K, Nieminen MS, *et al.* (1988). Serological evidence of an association of a novel chlamydia TWAR with chronic coronary heart disease and acute myocardial infarction. *Lancet* **2:** 963-6.

6. Saikku P, Leinonen M, Tenkanen L, *et al.* (1992). Chronic *C. pneumoniae* disease in Helsinki Heart Study. *Ann Intern Med* **116:** 273–8.

7. Juvonen J, Juvonen T, Laurila A, *et al.* (1998). Can degenerative aortic valve stenosis be related to persistent *Chlamydia pneumoniae* infection? *Ann Intern Med* **128:** 741–4.

8. Petersen E, Boman J, Persson K, *et al.* (1998). *Chlamydia pneumoniae* in human abdominal aortic aneurysms. *Eur J Vascular Endovascular Surgery* **15:** 138–42.

9. Kreiger JN, Riley DE, Roberts MC, Bergen RE. (1996) Prokaryotic DNA sequences in patients with chronic idiopathic prostatitis. *J Clin Microbiol* **34:** 3120–8.

10. Gerard HC, Branigan PJ, Schumacher HR Jr, *et al.* (1998). Synovial *C. trachomatis* in patients with reactive Reiter's syndrome are viable but show aberrant gene expressions. *J Rheumatol* **25:** 734–42.

11. Morrison RP. (1998). Persistent *C. trachomatis* infection: *in vitro* phenomenon or *in vivo* trigger of reactive arthritis? (Editorial) *J Rheumatol* **25:** 610–12.

12. Muller-Schoob JW, Wana S-P, Murgine J, *et al.* (1978). *C. trachomatis* as possible cause of peritonitis, perihepatitis in young women. *Br Med J* **1:** 1022–4.

13. Eschenvach DA. (1984). Sexually Transmited Diseases. New York: McGraw Hill, 633–8.

14. Shanahan D. (1990). Cloak and dagger – studies of chlamydial peritonitis in humans and mice. Paper read at meeting of the Medical Society for the Study of Venereal Disease, London. 30 November 1990.

15. Hillis SD, Coles FB, Lichfield B. *et al.* (1998). Doxycycline and azithromycin for prevention of chlamydial persistence or recurrence one month after treatment of women. A use-effectiveness study in public health. *Sex Trans Dis* **25;** 5–11.

16. Kaufpinen MJ, Saikku P, Kujala P. *et al.* (1996). Clinical picture of community acquired *Chlamydia pneumoniae* pneumonia requiring hospital treatment: a comparison between chlamydia and pneumococcal pneumonia. *Thorax* **51:** 185–90.

17. Munday PK. (1985). Persistent and recurrent NGU. In: Taylor-Robinson D. ed. *Clinical Problems in Sexually Transmitted Disease*. Dordrecht: Martinus Nijhof, 15–35.

18. Blythe MJ, Katz BP, Battergar BE *et al.* (1992). Recurrent genitourinary chlamydial infections in sexually active female adolescents. *J Pediatr* **121:** 487–93.

19. Dhar J, Arya OP, Timmins DJ. *et al.* (1992). The efficacy of azithromycin versus doxycycline in the treatment of non-gonococcal urethritis (abstract) *MSSVD Meeting,* Dublin 1992.

20. Bhattacharya MN, Morton RS. (1971). Long term triple tetracycline therapy in non-specific urethritis. *Br J Vener Dis* **147:** 266–9.

21. Hurst EW, Landquist JK, Melvin P. (1950). The therapy of experimental psittacosis and lymphogranuloma venereum. *Br J Pharm Chemother* **5:** 611–24.

22. Hurst EW, Landquist JK, Melvin P, *et al.* (1953). The therapy of experimental psittacosis and lymphogranuloma venereum. *Br J Pharm Chemother* **8:** 197–305.

23. Morton RS. (1983). A reappraisal of non-specific genital infection with reference to the work of the late Dr E Weston-Hurst. *Br J Vener Dis* **59:** 394–6.

24. Evans BA. (1978). The role of tetracyclines in the treatment of non-specific urethritis. *Br J Vener Dis* **54:** 107–11.

25. Woolley PD, Kinghorn GR, Talbot MD *et al.* (1990). Efficiency of combined metronidazole and triple tetracycline therapy in treatment of NGU. *Int J Sex Trans Dis AIDS* **1:** 35–7.

26. Evans BA. (1977). The role of tetracyclines in the treatment of non-specific urethritis. *Br J Vener Dis* **53:** 40–3.

27. Helmy N, Fowler W. (1975). Intensive and prolonged tetracycline therapy in non-specific urethritis. *Br J Vener Dis* **51:** 336–9.

28. Rosedale N. (1959). Female consorts of men with NGU. *Br J Vner Dis* **35:** 245–8.

29. Fitzgerald MR. (1984). Effect of epidemiological treatment of contacts in preventing recurrence of NGU. *Br J Vener Dis* **60:** 312–15.

30. Woolley PD, Wilson JD, Kinghorn GR. (1987). Epidemiological treatment of sexual contacts prevents recurrence of NGU. *Genitourin Med* **63:** 384–5.
31. Shamanesh M, Pandit PG, Pound R. (1996). Urethral lymphocyte isolations in non-gonococcal urethritis. *Genitourin Med* **72:** 362–4.
32. Cohen MS, Hoffman JF, Royce RA *et al.* (1997). Reduction of concentration of HIV-1 in semen after treatment of urethritis: implications for prevention of sexual transmission of HIV-1. *Lancet* **349:** 1863–73.
33. Atkins Ml, Carlin EM, Emery VC, *et al.* (1996). Fluctuations of HIV load in semen of HIV positive patients with newly acquired sexually transmitted diseases. *Br Med J* **313:** 341–2.
34. Leiberman D, Schoeffer F, Dolder I, *et al.* (1996). Multiple pathogens in adult patients admitted with community-acquired pneumonia: a one-year prospective study of 346 consecutive patients. *Thorax* **51:** 179–84.
35. Jackson LA, Nicholas LS, Hickbert SR, *et al.* (1999). Lack of association between first myocardial infarction and past use of erythromycin, tetracycline, and doxycycline. *Emerg Infect Dis* **5:** 281–4.
36. Gupta S, Leathens EW. Carrington D, *et al.* (1997). Elevated *C. pneumoniae* antibodies cardiovascular events, and azithromycin in male survivors of myocardial infection.*Circulation* **96:** 404–7.
37. Sinisalo J, Mattila K. Nieminen MS *et al.* (1998). The effect of prolonged doxycyline therapy on *Chlamydia pneumoniae* serological markers, coronary heart disease risk, and forearm based nitric oxide production. *J Antimicrobiol Chemother* **41:** 85–92.
38. Johnson JD, Hand WL, Francis JB *et al.* (1980). Antibiotic uptake by alveolar macrophages. *J Lab Clin Med* **95:** 429–39.
39. Morton RS, Kinghorn GR. (1999). Genitourinary chlamydial infection: a reappraisal and hypothesis. *Int J STD & AIDS.* **10:** 765–775.